Updates in Breast Reconstruction: Review from Evidence

Updates in Breast Reconstruction: Review from Evidence

Editors

Andrea Sisti
Roberto Cuomo

MDPI • Basel • Beijing • Wuhan • Barcelona • Belgrade • Manchester • Tokyo • Cluj • Tianjin

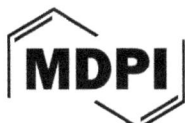

Editors
Andrea Sisti
Cleveland Clinic Ohio
USA

Roberto Cuomo
University of Siena
Italy

Editorial Office
MDPI
St. Alban-Anlage 66
4052 Basel, Switzerland

This is a reprint of articles from the Special Issue published online in the open access journal *Medicina* (ISSN 1010-660X) (available at: https://www.mdpi.com/journal/water/special_issues/hydraulics_numerical_methods).

For citation purposes, cite each article independently as indicated on the article page online and as indicated below:

LastName, A.A.; LastName, B.B.; LastName, C.C. Article Title. *Journal Name* **Year**, *Volume Number*, Page Range.

ISBN 978-3-0365-1110-8 (Hbk)
ISBN 978-3-0365-1111-5 (PDF)

© 2021 by the authors. Articles in this book are Open Access and distributed under the Creative Commons Attribution (CC BY) license, which allows users to download, copy and build upon published articles, as long as the author and publisher are properly credited, which ensures maximum dissemination and a wider impact of our publications.

The book as a whole is distributed by MDPI under the terms and conditions of the Creative Commons license CC BY-NC-ND.

Contents

About the Editors vii

Preface to "Updates in Breast Reconstruction: Review from Evidence" ix

Roberto Cuomo
Submuscular and Pre-pectoral ADM Assisted Immediate Breast Reconstruction: A Literature Review
Reprinted from: *Medicina* **2020**, *56*, 256, doi:10.3390/medicina56060256 1

Kristina Crawford and Matthew Endara
Lipotransfer Strategies and Techniques to Achieve Successful Breast Reconstruction in the Radiated Breast
Reprinted from: *Medicina* **2020**, *56*, 516, doi:10.3390/medicina56100516 13

Giovanni Papa, Andrea Frasca, Nadia Renzi, Chiara Stocco, Giuseppe Pizzolato, Vittorio Ramella and Zoran Marij Arnež
Protocol for Prevention and Monitoring of Surgical Site Infections in Implant-Based Breast Reconstruction: Preliminary Results
Reprinted from: *Medicina* **2021**, *57*, 151, doi:10.3390/medicina57020151 25

Jeong-Hoon Kim, Jin-Woo Park and Kyong-Je Woo
Prediction of the Ideal Implant Size Using 3-Dimensional Healthy Breast Volume in Unilateral Direct-to-Implant Breast Reconstruction
Reprinted from: *Medicina* **2020**, *56*, 498, doi:10.3390/medicina56100498 37

Jin-Woo Park, Jeong Hoon Kim and Kyong-Je Woo
Intraoperative Intercostal Nerve Block for Postoperative Pain Control in Pre-Pectoral versus Subpectoral Direct-To-Implant Breast Reconstruction: A Retrospective Study
Reprinted from: *Medicina* **2020**, *56*, 325, doi:10.3390/medicina56070325 47

David J. Restrepo, Maria T. Huayllani, Daniel Boczar, Andrea Sisti, Minh-Doan T. Nguyen, Jordan J. Cochuyt, Aaron C. Spaulding, Brian D. Rinker, Galen Perdikis and Antonio J. Forte
Disparities in Access to Autologous Breast Reconstruction
Reprinted from: *Medicina* **2020**, *56*, 281, doi:10.3390/medicina56060281 61

Andrea Sisti
Nipple–Areola Complex Reconstruction
Reprinted from: *Medicina* **2020**, *56*, 296, doi:10.3390/medicina56060296 71

About the Editors

Andrea Sisti is a Plastic Surgeon, with both clinical and research experience. He is now Craniofacial Surgery Fellow at the Department of Plastic Surgery, Cleveland Clinic Ohio (USA). Dr Sisti completed his Medical School at the University of Bologna (Italy) and his Plastic Surgery Residency at the University of Siena (Italy). Furthermore, he completed his first Residency in Family Medicine at University of Florence (Italy) from 2009 to 2012. He spent a year at Mayo Clinic Florida (USA) as Research Trainee and a year at Cleveland Clinic Ohio (USA) as a Visiting Researcher/Research Fellow.

Roberto Cuomo As a Specialist in Plastic Surgery Clinic at Santa Maria Alle Scotte Hospital, Dr Cuomo is one of the youngest Assistant Professors in his country. Dr. Cuomo's clinical practice is devoted to the care of patients after massive weight loss with breast health issues and for breast reconstruction. He has published novel surgical tips in reconstructive breast surgery to reduce pain and to improve cosmetic outcomes in breast reconstruction in international Journals. He has also authored book chapters indexed in the most common databases of peer-reviewed literature. Dr Cuomo is Member of SICPRE (Italian Society of Plastic, Reconstructive and Aesthetic Surgery), and AICPEO (Italian Association of Aesthetic Plastic Surgery of Obesity). He has given more than 50 oral presentations in national and international meetings, and is a member of the editorial panel of four international journals. Dr. Cuomo is constantly engaged in research into new techniques and technologies for regenerative surgery to improve the long-term results in breast surgery in cancer and post-bariatric patients.

Preface to "Updates in Breast Reconstruction: Review from Evidence"

Dear Colleagues,

Breast cancer treatment has changed dramatically in the last 50 years. The advancement of technologies and better patient management have made new strategies possible for breast reconstruction. Breast reconstruction is an integral part of "breast cancer treatment" in many countries. Many techniques have been introduced, and all of them have strengths and weaknesses that should be carefully investigated.

Furthermore, there is concern about different levels of access to the most advanced and expensive treatments for breast reconstruction due to social disparities.

The use of biomaterials, such as acellular dermal matrices, and microsurgical reconstruction represent a burden on health systems and are not accessible to everyone.

The final step of breast reconstruction is the nipple–areola complex reconstruction; this is a very important surgical procedure, for which many techniques have been described.

We believe that clarity is needed on these topics, based on scientific evidence. This Special Issue aims to capture the experience of world-class experts in breast cancer reconstruction.

Andrea Sisti, Roberto Cuomo
Editors

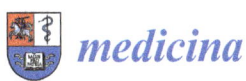

Article

Submuscular and Pre-pectoral ADM Assisted Immediate Breast Reconstruction: A Literature Review

Roberto Cuomo

Santa Maria Alle Scotte Hospital, Plastic and Reconstructive Surgery Unit, Department of Medicine, Surgery and Neuroscience, University of Siena, Mario Bracci Street, 53100 Siena, Italy; robertocuomo@outlook.com

Received: 7 April 2020; Accepted: 23 May 2020; Published: 26 May 2020

Abstract: *Background and objectives*: Breast cancer treatment has deeply changed in the last fifty years. Acellular dermal matrices (ADMs) were introduced for breast reconstruction, with encouraging results, but with conflicting reports too. The present paper aims to summarize the current data on breast reconstruction using acellular dermal matrices. *Materials and Methods*: We reviewed the literature regarding the use of ADM-assisted implant-based breast reconstruction. *Results*: The main techniques were analyzed and described. *Conclusions*: Several authors have recently reported positive results. Nevertheless, an increased complications' rate has been reported by other authors. Higher cost compared to not-ADM-assisted breast reconstruction is another concern.

Keywords: acellular dermal matrix; ADM; breast reconstruction; pre-pectoral; submuscular

1. Introduction

The use of acellular dermal matrix (ADM) for breast reconstruction was described by Salzberg in 2006 [1] and by Dieterich in 2015 [2,3]. Acellular dermal matrices (ADMs) are made from fetal bovine, porcine or human cadaver and represent a sort of scaffold that autologous cells can colonize [4,5].

Immediate breast reconstruction (IBR) received an important boost in popularity as a consequence of the advent of ADMs [2,6–19]. The use of ADMs showed encouraging results but conflicting reports as well [20–42]. ADMs-assisted breast reconstruction can be divided into pre-pectoral and submuscular. The present narrative review summarizes the current evidences on immediate breast reconstruction using ADM.

2. Materials and Methods

We performed a review of literature, starting from 2006, by searching on PubMed "acellular dermal matrix" and "breast reconstruction", focusing on surgical techniques, outcomes and complications' rate, in order to better understand the evidences on this topic.

3. Results

3.1. Acellular Dermal Matrix (ADM) and Breast Reconstruction

Immediate breast reconstruction (IBR) has radically changed the concept of breast cancer to the extent that a patient admitted to surgery for breast cancer is discharged without the impact of breast amputation.

The main advantages of IBR can be summarized as lower costs for the healthcare system (shorter healing time and fewer hospitalizations) and the elimination of tissue expansion time [43–47]. Despite this, several studies have reported high rates of complications linked to immediate breast reconstruction [2,7,48–51]. Many authors analyzed these aspects, underlining the safety of IBR and the good outcomes reached with careful patient selection and adherence to surgical techniques [2,52–63]. IBR has similar postoperative complications to delayed breast reconstructions with tissue expander and implant, although tissue expander/submuscular implant has been the most popular reconstruction strategy [43,44,64–67].

The American Society of Plastic Surgeons reported the use of ADMs in about 50% of breast reconstruction in 2012 [68], and these data were confirmed over time [69].

Recent research confirmed good outcomes for ADMs assisted IBR as underlined by Negeborn et al. [35,70] and Carminati et al. [21], with acceptable risks of infection. This risk is higher in obese patients [21]. Improved aesthetic outcomes following ADM use in tissue expander/implant-based breast reconstruction was assessed by Ibrahim et al. [71]. ADM may improve breast volume, placement and inframammary fold definition [72].

The main disadvantage of this kind of procedure is the high costs, as shown by Gravina et al. [24]. They analyzed the different characteristics of the main ADMs and their alternatives, underlining the good aesthetic outcomes and the benefits of single-stage procedures, but these aspects are balanced with high costs and an increased risk of infection and overall surgical complication [24].

Many authors agree that IBR received an important boost in popularity as a consequence of the advent of AMDs [2,6–18]. ADM-assisted breast reconstruction can be divided into submuscular and pre-pectoral.

3.2. Submuscular ADM-Assisted Breast Reconstruction

In submuscular breast reconstruction, the surgeon can place an ADM to cover the inferior pole of the implant [73–76]. This is helpful in the following situations:

(1) The breast has a good volume, and the surgeon needs to use an implant of adequate volume for immediate reconstruction, but the inferior pole of the implant cannot be completely covered by the Pectoralis Major [9,10,57,77,78].

(2) To prevent the need of major elevation of muscle, reducing postoperative pain [77,79–81].

Partial muscle coverage is important to obtain a more natural shape, releasing the constriction of the inferior aspect of pectoralis muscle but less coverage of prostheses in the lateral-inferior aspect can occur in some cases [77,82].

Lateral control of the implant position can be obtained by using Serratus or minimizing the lateral dissection during the mastectomy, but this may not be enough. In these cases, the use of an ADM allows surgeons to better control the stability of the breast implant both in immediate and delayed breast reconstruction [77,83–86].

The submuscular breast reconstruction performed using ADM to cover the lateral or the inferior pole of neo-breast is routinely referred to as dual-plane reconstruction (see Figure 1). The most common anti-aesthetic reports is the muscle retraction deformity; this can be avoided by suturing the ADM at the inferior border of the muscle, from the four to eight o'clock position [77,84,87].

Lateral sutures can be used between the skin flap and the chest wall to better close the dead space and improve the lateral contour, but the skin thickness should be carefully evaluated, in order to avoid quilting sutures [8,64,88–92].

Many authors agree that this kind of reconstruction has excellent long-term cosmetic results; the main unexpected event is the distortion or the movement of the implant with flexion of the muscle. Compared to pre-pectoral reconstruction, it is less expensive and can lead to better coverage of the upper pole of the breast. Nevertheless, it is burdened by the risk of upper migration of the implant and more pain due to muscle detachment [2,7,77,83,89–91].

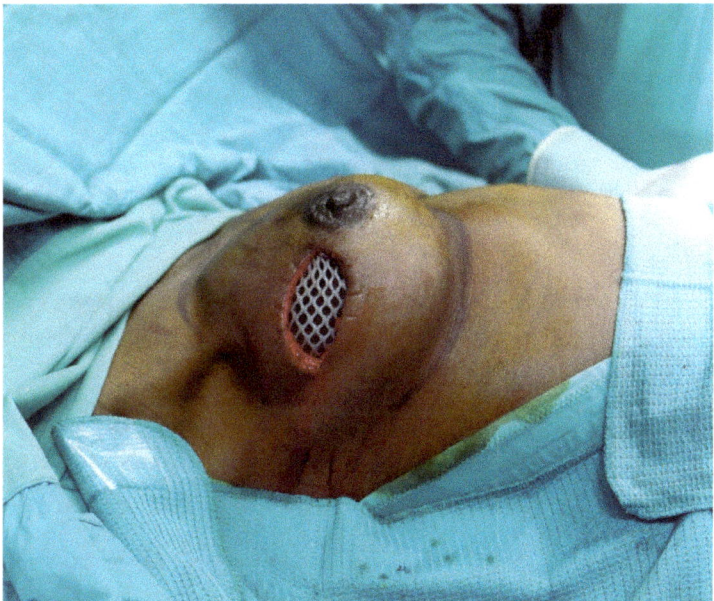

Figure 1. Meshed ADM used to cover the inferolateral aspect of the implant in submuscular breast reconstruction. ADM: Acellular dermal matrix.

3.3. Pre-Pectoral ADM-Assisted Breast Reconstruction

The concept of pre-pectoral breast reconstruction (see Figure 2) can be considered as the "evolution" of breast reconstruction in terms of "tissue sparing": As nipple-skin sparing mastectomy for the oncologic surgery, pre-pectoral breast reconstruction focuses on sparing the Pectoralis Major Muscle. ADM has a key role in this kind of procedure because it wraps (at least in the front) the implant for a complete integration in the host [93,94].

Pre-pectoral breast reconstruction was suggested in those cases where implants less than 500 cc were requested [95]. Actually, this indication has been modified, and some authors describe pre-pectoral breast reconstruction with implants over 600 cc [77].

Many authors choose the pre-pectoral breast reconstruction because the submuscular placement of the implant can lead to a result described as "contrived breast" [82,91,95,96]. This aspect is relevant and linked to a loss of muscle function; many authors, in fact, underline that patients, in particular after tissue expansion, need physiotherapy. The muscle-spearing breast reconstruction was proposed by many authors over time.

In 2013, Cheng proposed the treatment of capsular contracture using an ADM; he did not perform pre-pectoral reconstruction, but removed the contracted capsule and put ADM to cover the anterior aspect of the implant on 16 breasts. He reported only one infection by coagulase negative Staphylococcus and Mycobacterium fortuitum [97]. The reduction of incidence in capsular contracture using ADMs was underlined in time by Lardi et al., in 2017 [30], and confirmed by Liu et al., with a meta-analysis in 2020 [33].

Becker et al. (2015) reported the experience on 62 breasts covering the anterior aspect of saline implant with an ADM sutured to the muscle. The complications reported were three flap necrosis, one seroma, one infection, one hematoma and two capsular contractures [98].

In 2017, Berna firstly proposed a complete ADM coverage of the implant [93]; the implant stability was guaranteed by suturing the implant and its "envelope" to the muscle. On 100 reconstructions with this procedure, Vidya et al. underlined two hematoma, three dehiscence, one necrosis, five seromas and two implant losses [95].

The main purpose of pre-pectoral reconstruction is to save the function of Pectoralis Major, decreasing the postoperative pain and reducing the follow-up time. Other advantages are represented by minor risk in the upper migration of the implant and a better breast projection [99,100].

The main disadvantages are the high costs of these devices (which are to be added to the cost of breast implants) and the higher risk of symmastia, the rippling and an irregularity of the highest limit of the upper pole of the breast and the high risk of seroma. Several authors suggest not removing the drains until finding a maximum of 30cc for three consecutive days [18,77,101].

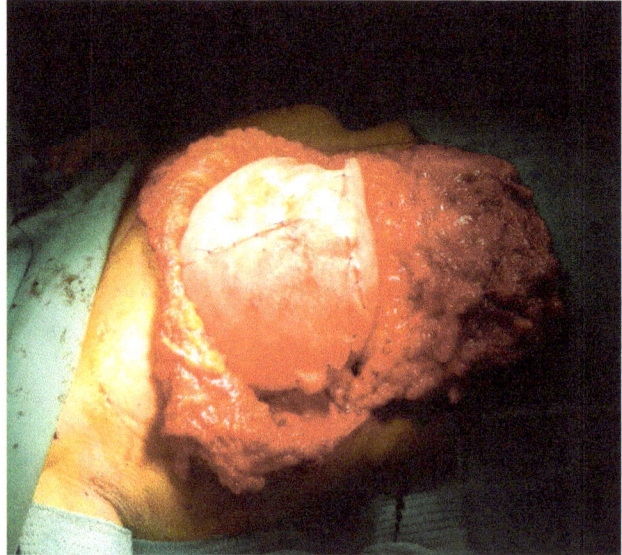

Figure 2. ADM-assisted pre-pectoral breast reconstruction with vertical scar.

The dimpling of the upper pole of the breast occurs due to the thinning of the subcutaneous tissue and can be avoided with lipofilling [102] or leaving 1 cm of subcutaneous fat in selected cases [103] or harvesting tissue from the muscle [104].

3.4. Complications and Outcomes

Tasoulis et al. observed that ADM-assisted breast reconstruction reduces the complications' rate [105]. Onesti et al. observed that the use of ADM reduces the inflammatory response, along with the likelihood of capsular contracture [36].

On the other hand, Lohmander et al. [106] observed that immediate IBR with ADM carried a risk of implant loss equal to conventional IBR without ADM, but was associated with more adverse outcomes, requiring surgical intervention, through an open-label, multicenter, randomized, controlled trial on 135 women. Antony et al. [107]. observed that acellular human dermis is useful in immediate tissue expander reconstruction but can lead to an increased risk of complications (seroma and reconstructive failure).

The literature data show that the complications' rate is similar for subcutaneous and submuscular reconstruction ADM assisted, without statistical significance for major adverse events (explantation, wide infections, Baker grade III or IV contracture, and complete nipple–areola complex necrosis) [22]. Overall, the most described complications for ADMs-assisted reconstruction are seroma (up to 9% of cases), explantation (up to 6.5%) and partial nipple–areola complex (NAC) necrosis (up to 5.3%) [2,37,65,83,108–112].

In 2017, Kim and Bang linked the use of ADM and the mastectomy flap necrosis [28]. Powell-Brett and Goh [113] reported 10.4% cases of skin necrosis in a study with ADM-assisted immediate breast reconstruction.

This last complication should be interpreted as follows: It can occur (in some cases) for tissue ischemia during the cancer removing and the implant. Intraoperative tools to evaluate NAC viability can lower this complication's rate, but these devices are expensive, time-consuming and not available in all centers [41,114–116].

The pre-pectoral breast reconstruction is burdened by the following patient complaints: rippling (up to 4.5%) and visible implants (4.3%). The submuscular breast reconstruction is burdened by postoperative pain with significant impact on daily activities (5%), implant deformity and less-natural cosmetic outcomes (until 7%) [6,93,108,117–124]. Onesti et al. suggested a modified technique in obesity patients with large breasts, using a dermal flap to cover the ADM-implant in the pre-pectoral plane, in order to improve the outcomes. Obesity and smoking are always linked to a higher risk of complications [125–127].

4. Conclusions

Pre-pectoral and submuscular breast reconstruction with the use of ADMs have no significant difference in complication rate. Particular care must be taken for seroma formation. Obesity and smoking are linked to higher risks of complication. The cost/benefit ratio should be carefully reviewed.

Funding: This research received no external funding.

Conflicts of Interest: The author declares no conflict of interest.

References

1. Salzberg, C.A. Nonexpansive immediate breast reconstruction using human acellular tissue matrix graft (AlloDerm). *Ann. Plast. Surg.* **2006**, *57*, 1–5. [CrossRef] [PubMed]
2. Bertozzi, N.; Pesce, M.; Santi, P.; Raposio, E. One-Stage Immediate Breast Reconstruction: A Concise Review. *Biomed. Res. Int.* **2017**. [CrossRef] [PubMed]
3. Dieterich, M.; Angres, J.; Stubert, J.; Stachs, A.; Reimer, T.; Gerber, B. Patient-Reported Outcomes in Implant-Based Breast Reconstruction Alone or in Combination with a Titanium-Coated Polypropylene Mesh—A Detailed Analysis of the BREAST-Q and Overview of the Literature. *Geburtshilfe Frauenheilkd.* **2015**, *75*, 692–701. [CrossRef] [PubMed]
4. Butler, C.E.; Selber, J.C. Discussion: The use of acellular dermal matrix in immediate two-stage tissue expander breast reconstruction. *Plast. Reconstr. Surg.* **2012**, *129*, 1059–1060. [CrossRef]
5. Margulies, I.G.; Salzberg, C.A. The use of acellular dermal matrix in breast reconstruction: Evolution of techniques over 2 decades. *Gland Surg.* **2019**, *8*, 3–10. [CrossRef] [PubMed]
6. Basta, M.N.; Gerety, P.A.; Serletti, J.M.; Kovach, S.J.; Fischer, J.P. A Systematic Review and Head-to-Head Meta-Analysis of Outcomes following Direct-to-Implant versus Conventional Two-Stage Implant Reconstruction. *Plast. Reconstr. Surg.* **2015**, *136*, 1135–1144. [CrossRef] [PubMed]
7. Colwell, A.S.; Damjanovic, B.; Zahedi, B.; Medford-Davis, L.; Hertl, C.; Austen, W.G., Jr. Retrospective review of 331 consecutive immediate single-stage implant reconstructions with acellular dermal matrix: Indications, complications, trends, and costs. *Plast. Reconstr. Surg.* **2011**, *128*, 1170–1178. [CrossRef]
8. Cordeiro, P.G. Discussion: Focus on technique: Two-stage implant-based breast reconstruction. *Plast. Reconstr. Surg.* **2012**, *130*, 116S–117S. [CrossRef]
9. Cordeiro, P.G.; McCarthy, C.M. A single surgeon's 12-year experience with tissue expander/implant breast reconstruction: Part II. An analysis of long-term complications, aesthetic outcomes, and patient satisfaction. *Plast. Reconstr. Surg.* **2006**, *118*, 832–839. [CrossRef]
10. Cordeiro, P.G.; McCarthy, C.M. A single surgeon's 12-year experience with tissue expander/implant breast reconstruction: Part I. A prospective analysis of early complications. *Plast. Reconstr. Surg.* **2006**, *118*, 825–831. [CrossRef]

11. Glasberg, S.B. The Economics of Prepectoral Breast Reconstruction. *Plast. Reconstr. Surg.* **2017**, *140*, 49S–52S. [CrossRef] [PubMed]
12. Glasberg, S.B.; Light, D. AlloDerm and Strattice in breast reconstruction: A comparison and techniques for optimizing outcomes. *Plast. Reconstr. Surg.* **2012**, *129*, 1223–1233. [CrossRef] [PubMed]
13. Lennox, P.A.; Bovill, E.S.; Macadam, S.A. Evidence-Based Medicine: Alloplastic Breast Reconstruction. *Plast. Reconstr. Surg.* **2017**, *140*, 94e–108e. [CrossRef]
14. Lindford, A.J.; Meretoja, T.J.; von Smitten, K.A.; Jahkola, T.A. Skin-sparing mastectomy and immediate breast reconstruction in the management of locally recurrent breast cancer. *Ann. Surg. Oncol.* **2010**, *17*, 1669–1674. [CrossRef] [PubMed]
15. Meretoja, T.J.; von Smitten, K.A.; Kuokkanen, H.O.; Suominen, S.H.; Jahkola, T.A. Complications of skin-sparing mastectomy followed by immediate breast reconstruction: A prospective randomized study comparing high-frequency radiosurgery with conventional diathermy. *Ann. Plast. Surg.* **2008**, *60*, 24–28. [CrossRef] [PubMed]
16. Sbitany, H.; Lee, K.R. Optimizing Outcomes in 2-Stage Prepectoral Breast Reconstruction Utilizing Round Form-Stable Implants. *Plast. Reconstr. Surg.* **2019**, *144*, 43S–50S. [CrossRef] [PubMed]
17. Srinivasa, D.R.; Holland, M.; Sbitany, H. Optimizing perioperative strategies to maximize success with prepectoral breast reconstruction. *Gland Surg.* **2019**, *8*, 19–26. [CrossRef]
18. Vidya, R.; Berna, G.; Sbitany, H.; Nahabedian, M.; Becker, H.; Reitsamer, R.; Rancati, A.; Macmillan, D.; Cawthorn, S. Prepectoral implant-based breast reconstruction: A joint consensus guide from UK, European and USA breast and plastic reconstructive surgeons. *Ecancermedicalscience* **2019**, *13*, 927. [CrossRef]
19. Sisti, A.; Huayllani, M.T.; Boczar, D.; Restrepo, D.J.; Spaulding, A.C.; Emmanuel, G.; Bagaria, S.P.; McLaughlin, S.A.; Parker, A.S.; Forte, A.J. Breast cancer in women: A descriptive analysis of the national cancer database. *Acta Biomed.* **2020**, *91*, 332–341. [CrossRef]
20. Ball, J.F.; Huayllani, M.T.; Boczar, D.; Restrepo, D.J.; Spaulding, A.C.; Emmanuel, G.; Bagaria, S.P.; McLaughlin, S.A.; Parker, A.S.; Forte, A.J. A direct comparison of porcine (Strattice) and bovine (Surgimend) acellular dermal matrices in implant-based immediate breast reconstruction. *JPRAS* **2017**, *70*, 1076–1082. [CrossRef] [PubMed]
21. Carminati, M.; Sempf, D.; Bonfirraro, P.P.; Devalle, L.; Verga, M.; Righi, B.; Mevio, G.; Leone, F.; Fenaroli, P.; Robotti, E. Immediate Implant-based Breast Reconstruction with Acellular Dermal Matrix Compared with Tissue-expander Breast Reconstruction: Rate of Infection. *Plast. Reconstr. Surg. Glob. Open* **2018**, *6*, e1949. [CrossRef] [PubMed]
22. Chandarana, M.; Harries, S.; National Braxon Audit Study, G. Multicentre study of prepectoral breast reconstruction using acellular dermal matrix. *BJS Open* **2020**, *4*, 71–77. [CrossRef] [PubMed]
23. Eichler, C.; Schulz, C.; Vogt, N.; Warm, M. The Use of Acellular Dermal Matrices (ADM) in Breast Reconstruction: A Review. *Surg. Technol. Int.* **2017**, *31*, 53–60. [PubMed]
24. Gravina, P.R.; Pettit, R.W.; Davis, M.J.; Winocour, S.J.; Selber, J.C. Evidence for the Use of Acellular Dermal Matrix in Implant-Based Breast Reconstruction. *Semin. Plast. Surg.* **2019**, *33*, 229–235. [CrossRef] [PubMed]
25. Greig, H.; Roller, J.; Ziaziaris, W.; Van Laeken, N. A retrospective review of breast reconstruction outcomes comparing AlloDerm and DermaCELL. *JPRAS Open* **2019**, *22*, 19–26. [CrossRef] [PubMed]
26. Hinchcliff, K.M.; Orbay, H.; Busse, B.K.; Charvet, H.; Kaur, M.; Sahar, D.E. Comparison of two cadaveric acellular dermal matrices for immediate breast reconstruction: A prospective randomized trial. *JPRAS* **2017**, *70*, 568–576. [CrossRef]
27. Kim, A.; Jung, J.H.; Choi, Y.L.; Pyon, J.K. Capsule biopsy of acellular dermal matrix (ADM) to predict future capsular contracture in two-stage prosthetic breast reconstruction. *JPRAS* **2019**, *72*, 1576–1606. [CrossRef]
28. Kim, S.Y.; Bang, S.I. Impact of Acellular Dermal Matrix (ADM) Use under Mastectomy Flap Necrosis on Perioperative Outcomes of Prosthetic Breast Reconstruction. *Aesthet. Plast. Surg.* **2017**, *41*, 275–281. [CrossRef]
29. Knabben, L.; Kanagalingam, G.; Imboden, S.; Gunthert, A.R. Acellular Dermal Matrix (Permacol®) for Heterologous Immediate Breast Reconstruction after Skin-Sparing Mastectomy in Patients with Breast Cancer: A Single-Institution Experience and a Review of the Literature. *Front. Med.* **2016**, *3*, 72. [CrossRef] [PubMed]
30. Lardi, A.M.; Ho-Asjoe, M.; Junge, K.; Farhadi, J. Capsular contracture in implant based breast reconstruction-the effect of porcine acellular dermal matrix. *Gland Surg.* **2017**, *6*, 49–56. [CrossRef]

31. Lee, C.U.; Bobr, A.; Torres-Mora, J. Radiologic-Pathologic Correlation: Acellular Dermal Matrix (Alloderm®) Used in Breast Reconstructive Surgery. *J. Clin. Imaging Sci.* **2017**, *7*, 13. [CrossRef] [PubMed]
32. Lee, J.S.; Kim, J.S.; Lee, J.H.; Lee, J.W.; Lee, J.; Park, H.Y.; Yang, J.D. Prepectoral breast reconstruction with complete implant coverage using double-crossed acellular dermal matrixs. *Gland Surg.* **2019**, *8*, 748–757. [CrossRef] [PubMed]
33. Liu, J.; Hou, J.; Li, Z.; Wang, B.; Sun, J. Efficacy of Acellular Dermal Matrix in Capsular Contracture of Implant-Based Breast Reconstruction: A Single-Arm Meta-analysis. *Aesthet. Plast. Surg.* **2020**. [CrossRef] [PubMed]
34. Mendenhall, S.D.; Anderson, L.A.; Ying, J.; Boucher, K.M.; Neumayer, L.A.; Agarwal, J.P. The BREASTrial Stage II: ADM Breast Reconstruction Outcomes from Definitive Reconstruction to 3 Months Postoperative. *Plast. Reconstr. Surg. Glob. Open* **2017**, *5*, e1209. [CrossRef] [PubMed]
35. Negenborn, V.L.; Dikmans, R.E.G.; Bouman, M.B.; Wilschut, J.A.; Mullender, M.G.; Salzberg, C.A. Patient-reported Outcomes after ADM-assisted Implant-based Breast Reconstruction: A Cross-sectional Study. *Plast. Reconstr. Surg. Glob. Open* **2018**, *6*, e1654. [CrossRef] [PubMed]
36. Onesti, M.G.; Di Taranto, G.; Ribuffo, D.; Scuderi, N. ADM-assisted prepectoral breast reconstruction and skin reduction mastectomy: Expanding the indications for subcutaneous reconstruction. *JPRAS* **2019**. [CrossRef]
37. Paprottka, F.J.; Krezdorn, N.; Sorg, H.; Konneker, S.; Bontikous, S.; Robertson, I.; Schlett, C.L.; Dohse, N.K.; Hebebrand, D. Evaluation of Complication Rates after Breast Surgery Using Acellular Dermal Matrix: Median Follow-Up of Three Years. *Plast. Surg. Int.* **2017**, *2017*, 1283735. [CrossRef]
38. Singla, A.; Singla, A.; Lai, E.; Caminer, D. Subcutaneously Placed Breast Implants after a Skin-Sparing Mastectomy: Do We Always Need ADM? *Plast. Reconstr. Surg. Glob. Open* **2017**, *5*, e1371. [CrossRef]
39. Tsay, C.; Zhu, V.; Sturrock, T.; Shah, A.; Kwei, S. A 3D Mammometric Comparison of Implant-Based Breast Reconstruction with and Without Acellular Dermal Matrix (ADM). *Aesthet. Plast. Surg.* **2018**, *42*, 49–58. [CrossRef]
40. Vela-Lasagabaster, A.; Benito-Duque, P.; Ordonez-Maygua, J. Breast Prosthetic Reconstruction: Tips and Tricks on ADM Position. *Aesthet. Plast. Surg.* **2019**, *43*, 559–561. [CrossRef]
41. Zenn, M.; Venturi, M.; Pittman, T.; Spear, S.; Gurtner, G.; Robb, G.; Mesbahi, A.; Dayan, J. Optimizing Outcomes of Postmastectomy Breast Reconstruction with Acellular Dermal Matrix: A Review of Recent Clinical Data. *Eplasty* **2017**, *17*, e18. [PubMed]
42. Chao, A.H. A Review of the Use of Acellular Dermal Matrices in Postmastectomy Immediate Breast Reconstruction. *Plast. Surg. Nurs.* **2015**, *35*, 131–134. [CrossRef] [PubMed]
43. Frey, J.D.; Salibian, A.A.; Karp, N.S.; Choi, M. Implant-Based Breast Reconstruction: Hot Topics, Controversies, and New Directions. *Plast. Reconstr. Surg.* **2019**, *143*, 404e–416e. [CrossRef]
44. Frey, J.D.; Salibian, A.A.; Levine, J.P.; Karp, N.S.; Choi, M. Evolution of the Surgical Technique for "Breast in a Day" Direct-to-Implant Breast Reconstruction: Transitioning from Dual-Plane to Prepectoral Implant Placement. *Plast. Reconstr. Surg.* **2020**, *145*, 647e–648e. [CrossRef] [PubMed]
45. Krishnan, N.M.; Fischer, J.P.; Basta, M.N.; Nahabedian, M.Y. Is Single-Stage Prosthetic Reconstruction Cost Effective? A Cost-Utility Analysis for the Use of Direct-to-Implant Breast Reconstruction Relative to Expander-Implant Reconstruction in Postmastectomy Patients. *Plast. Reconstr. Surg.* **2016**, *138*, 537–547. [CrossRef] [PubMed]
46. Krishnan, N.M.; Purnell, C.; Nahabedian, M.Y.; Freed, G.L.; Nigriny, J.F.; Rosen, J.M.; Rosson, G.D. The cost effectiveness of the DIEP flap relative to the muscle-sparing TRAM flap in postmastectomy breast reconstruction. *Plast. Reconstr. Surg.* **2015**, *135*, 948–958. [CrossRef] [PubMed]
47. Salibian, A.A.; Frey, J.D.; Choi, M.; Karp, N.S. Subcutaneous Implant-based Breast Reconstruction with Acellular Dermal Matrix/Mesh: A Systematic Review. *Plast. Reconstr. Surg. Glob. Open* **2016**, *4*, e1139. [CrossRef]
48. Delgado, J.F.; Garcia-Guilarte, R.F.; Palazuelo, M.R.; Mendez, J.I.; Perez, C.C. Immediate breast reconstruction with direct, anatomic, gel-cohesive, extra-projection prosthesis: 400 cases. *Plast. Reconstr. Surg.* **2010**, *125*, 1599–1605. [CrossRef]
49. Gschwantler-Kaulich, D.; Schrenk, P.; Bjelic-Radisic, V.; Unterrieder, K.; Leser, C.; Fink-Retter, A.; Salama, M.; Singer, C. Mesh versus acellular dermal matrix in immediate implant-based breast reconstruction—A prospective randomized trial. *Eur. J. Surg. Oncol.* **2016**, *42*, 665–671. [CrossRef]

50. Salzberg, C.A.; Ashikari, A.Y.; Koch, R.M.; Chabner-Thompson, E. An 8-year experience of direct-to-implant immediate breast reconstruction using human acellular dermal matrix (AlloDerm). *Plast. Reconstr. Surg.* **2011**, *127*, 514–524. [CrossRef]
51. Agusti, A.; Ward, A.; Montgomery, C.; Mohammed, K.; Gui, G.P. Aesthetic and oncologic outcomes after one-stage immediate breast reconstruction using a permanent biodimensional expandable implant. *J. Plast. Reconstr. Aesthet. Surg.* **2016**, *69*, 211–220. [CrossRef]
52. Bailey, C.R.; Ogbuagu, O.; Baltodano, P.A.; Simjee, U.F.; Manahan, M.A.; Cooney, D.S.; Jacobs, L.K.; Tsangaris, T.N.; Cooney, C.M.; Rosson, G.D. Quality-of-Life Outcomes Improve with Nipple-Sparing Mastectomy and Breast Reconstruction. *Plast. Reconstr. Surg.* **2017**, *140*, 219–226. [CrossRef] [PubMed]
53. Bailey, M.H.; Smith, J.W.; Casas, L.; Johnson, P.; Serra, E.; de la Fuente, R.; Sullivan, M.; Scanlon, E.F. Immediate breast reconstruction: Reducing the risks. *Plast. Reconstr. Surg.* **1989**, *83*, 845–851. [CrossRef] [PubMed]
54. Fischer, J.P.; Cleveland, E.C.; Nelson, J.A.; Kovach, S.J.; Serletti, J.M.; Wu, L.C.; Kanchwala, S. Breast reconstruction in the morbidly obese patient: Assessment of 30-day complications using the 2005 to 2010 National Surgical Quality Improvement Program data sets. *Plast. Reconstr. Surg.* **2013**, *132*, 750–761. [CrossRef] [PubMed]
55. Fischer, J.P.; Wes, A.M.; Tuggle, C.T.; Serletti, J.M.; Wu, L.C. Risk analysis and stratification of surgical morbidity after immediate breast reconstruction. *J. Am. Coll. Surg.* **2013**, *217*, 780–787. [CrossRef]
56. Fischer, J.P.; Wes, A.M.; Tuggle, C.T.; Serletti, J.M., 3rd; Wu, L.C. Risk analysis of early implant loss after immediate breast reconstruction: A review of 14,585 patients. *J. Am. Coll. Surg.* **2013**, *217*, 983–990. [CrossRef]
57. Hvilsom, G.B.; Friis, S.; Frederiksen, K.; Steding-Jessen, M.; Henriksen, T.F.; Lipworth, L.; McLaughlin, J.K.; Elberg, J.J.; Damsgaard, T.E.; Holmich, L.R. The clinical course of immediate breast implant reconstruction after breast cancer. *Acta Oncol.* **2011**, *50*, 1045–1052. [CrossRef]
58. Hvilsom, G.B.; Holmich, L.R.; Frederiksen, K.; Steding-Jessen, M.; Friis, S.; Dalton, S.O. Socioeconomic position and breast reconstruction in Danish women. *Acta Oncol.* **2011**, *50*, 265–273. [CrossRef]
59. Hvilsom, G.B.; Holmich, L.R.; Steding-Jessen, M.; Frederiksen, K.; Henriksen, T.F.; Lipworth, L.; McLaughlin, J.; Elberg, J.J.; Damsgaard, T.E.; Friis, S. Delayed breast implant reconstruction: Is radiation therapy associated with capsular contracture or reoperations? *Ann. Plast. Surg.* **2012**, *68*, 246–252. [CrossRef]
60. Hvilsom, G.B.; Holmich, L.R.; Steding-Jessen, M.; Frederiksen, K.; Henriksen, T.F.; Lipworth, L.; McLaughlin, J.K.; Elberg, J.J.; Damsgaard, T.E.; Friis, S. Delayed breast implant reconstruction: A 10-year prospective study. *J. Plast. Reconstr. Aesthet. Surg.* **2011**, *64*, 1466–1474. [CrossRef]
61. Jansen, L.A.; Macadam, S.A. The use of AlloDerm in postmastectomy alloplastic breast reconstruction: Part I. A systematic review. *Plast. Reconstr. Surg.* **2011**, *127*, 2232–2244. [CrossRef]
62. Jansen, L.A.; Macadam, S.A. The use of AlloDerm in postmastectomy alloplastic breast reconstruction: Part II. A cost analysis. *Plast. Reconstr. Surg.* **2011**, *127*, 2245–2254. [CrossRef]
63. Menez, T.; Michot, A.; Tamburino, S.; Weigert, R.; Pinsolle, V. Multicenter evaluation of quality of life and patient satisfaction after breast reconstruction, a long-term retrospective study. *Ann. Chir. Plast. Esthet.* **2018**, *63*, 126–133. [CrossRef]
64. Cemal, Y.; Albornoz, C.R.; Disa, J.J.; McCarthy, C.M.; Mehrara, B.J.; Pusic, A.L.; Cordeiro, P.G.; Matros, E. A paradigm shift in U.S. breast reconstruction: Part 2. The influence of changing mastectomy patterns on reconstructive rate and method. *Plast. Reconstr. Surg.* **2013**, *131*, 320e–326e. [CrossRef]
65. Cuomo, R.; Nisi, G.; Grimaldi, L.; Brandi, C.; D'Aniello, C. Silicone breast implants and echocardiographic interactions: A brand new study. *Indian J. Plast. Surg.* **2016**, *49*, 430–431. [CrossRef]
66. Hirsch, E.M.; Seth, A.K.; Dumanian, G.A.; Kim, J.Y.; Mustoe, T.A.; Galiano, R.D.; Fine, N.A. Outcomes of immediate tissue expander breast reconstruction followed by reconstruction of choice in the setting of postmastectomy radiation therapy. *Ann. Plast. Surg.* **2014**, *72*, 274–278. [CrossRef]
67. Hirsch, E.M.; Seth, A.K.; Fine, N.A. Outcomes of immediate tissue expander breast reconstruction followed by reconstruction of choice in the setting of postmastectomy radiation therapy: Reply. *Ann. Plast. Surg.* **2015**, *74*, 271–272. [CrossRef]
68. 2012 Plastic Surgery Statistics Report. Available online: https://www.plasticsurgery.org/news/plastic-surgery-statistics?sub=2012+Plastic+Surgery+Statistics (accessed on 26 May 2020).
69. 2018 Plastic Surgery Statistics Report. Available online: https://www.plasticsurgery.org/news/plastic-surgery-statistics (accessed on 26 May 2020).

70. Negenborn, V.L.; Smit, J.M.; Dikmans, R.E.G.; Winters, H.A.H.; Twisk, J.W.R.; Ruhe, P.Q.; Mureau, M.A.M.; Tuinder, S.; Eltahir, Y.; Posch, N.A.S.; et al. Short-term cost-effectiveness of one-stage implant-based breast reconstruction with an acellular dermal matrix versus two-stage expander-implant reconstruction from a multicentre randomized clinical trial. *Br. J. Surg.* **2019**, *106*, 586–595. [CrossRef]
71. Ibrahim, A.M.; Koolen, P.G.; Ganor, O.; Markarian, M.K.; Tobias, A.M.; Lee, B.T.; Lin, S.J.; Mureau, M.A. Does acellular dermal matrix really improve aesthetic outcome in tissue expander/implant-based breast reconstruction? *Aesthet. Plast. Surg.* **2015**, *39*, 359–368. [CrossRef]
72. Nguyen, K.T.; Mioton, L.M.; Smetona, J.T.; Seth, A.K.; Kim, J.Y. Esthetic Outcomes of ADM-Assisted Expander-Implant Breast Reconstruction. *Eplasty* **2012**, *12*, e58.
73. Ho, A.L.; Klassen, A.F.; Cano, S.; Scott, A.M.; Pusic, A.L. Optimizing patient-centered care in breast reconstruction: The importance of preoperative information and patient-physician communication. *Plast. Reconstr. Surg.* **2013**, *132*, 212e–220e. [CrossRef]
74. Ho, A.L.; Tyldesley, S.; Macadam, S.A.; Lennox, P.A. Skin-sparing mastectomy and immediate autologous breast reconstruction in locally advanced breast cancer patients: A UBC perspective. *Ann. Surg. Oncol.* **2012**, *19*, 892–900. [CrossRef]
75. Ho, G.; Nguyen, T.J.; Shahabi, A.; Hwang, B.H.; Chan, L.S.; Wong, A.K. A systematic review and meta-analysis of complications associated with acellular dermal matrix-assisted breast reconstruction. *Ann. Plast. Surg.* **2012**, *68*, 346–356. [CrossRef]
76. Tom, L.; Broer, N.; Hoang, D.; Narayan, D. Novel use of acellularized dermis for breast reconstruction. *Plast. Reconstr. Surg.* **2011**, *128*, 31e–33e. [CrossRef]
77. Colwell, A.S.; Taylor, E.M. Recent Advances in Implant-Based Breast Reconstruction. *Plast. Reconstr. Surg.* **2020**, *145*, 421e–432e. [CrossRef]
78. Elliott, L.F.; Hartrampf, C.R., Jr. Breast reconstruction: Progress in the past decade. *World J. Surg.* **1990**, *14*, 763–775. [CrossRef]
79. Cuomo, R.; Zerini, I.; Botteri, G.; Barberi, L.; Nisi, G.; D'Aniello, C. Postsurgical pain related to breast implant: Reduction with lipofilling procedure. *In Vivo* **2014**, *28*, 993–996.
80. Juhl, A.A.; Christensen, S.; Zachariae, R.; Damsgaard, T.E. Unilateral breast reconstruction after mastectomy—Patient satisfaction, aesthetic outcome and quality of life. *Acta Oncol.* **2017**, *56*, 225–231. [CrossRef]
81. Juhl, A.A.; Damsgaard, T.E.; O'Connor, M.; Christensen, S.; Zachariae, R. Personality Traits as Predictors of Quality of Life and Body Image after Breast Reconstruction. *Plast. Reconstr. Surg. Glob. Open* **2017**, *5*, e1341. [CrossRef]
82. Breuing, K.H.; Colwell, A.S. Immediate breast tissue expander-implant reconstruction with inferolateral AlloDerm hammock and postoperative radiation: A preliminary report. *Eplasty* **2009**, *9*, e16.
83. Colwell, A.S.; Tessler, O.; Lin, A.M.; Liao, E.; Winograd, J.; Cetrulo, C.L.; Tang, R.; Smith, B.L.; Austen, W.G., Jr. Breast reconstruction following nipple-sparing mastectomy: Predictors of complications, reconstruction outcomes, and 5-year trends. *Plast. Reconstr. Surg.* **2014**, *133*, 496–506. [CrossRef]
84. Margulies, I.G.; Zoghbi, Y.; Jacobs, J.; Cate, S.P.; Salzberg, C.A. Direct to implant breast reconstruction: Visualized technique. *Gland Surg.* **2019**, *8*, S247–S250. [CrossRef]
85. Salzberg, C.A.; Ashikari, A.Y.; Berry, C.; Hunsicker, L.M. Acellular Dermal Matrix-Assisted Direct-to-Implant Breast Reconstruction and Capsular Contracture: A 13-Year Experience. *Plast. Reconstr. Surg.* **2016**, *138*, 329–337. [CrossRef]
86. Scheflan, M.; Colwell, A.S. Tissue Reinforcement in Implant-based Breast Reconstruction. *Plast. Reconstr. Surg. Glob. Open* **2014**, *2*, e192. [CrossRef]
87. Maisel Lotan, A.; Ben Yehuda, D.; Allweis, T.M.; Scheflan, M. Comparative Study of Meshed and Nonmeshed Acellular Dermal Matrix in Immediate Breast Reconstruction. *Plast. Reconstr. Surg.* **2019**, *144*, 1045–1053. [CrossRef]
88. Nelson, J.A.; Allen, R.J., Jr.; Polanco, T.; Shamsunder, M.; Patel, A.R.; McCarthy, C.M.; Matros, E.; Dayan, J.H.; Disa, J.J.; Cordeiro, P.G.; et al. Long-term Patient-reported Outcomes Following Postmastectomy Breast Reconstruction: An 8-year Examination of 3268 Patients. *Ann. Surg.* **2019**, *270*, 473–483. [CrossRef]
89. Baxter, R.A. Update on the split-muscle technique for breast augmentation: Prevention and correction of animation distortion and double-bubble deformity. *Aesthet. Plast. Surg.* **2011**, *35*, 426–429. [CrossRef]

90. Baxter, R.A. Long-term Follow-up with AlloDerm in Breast Reconstruction. *Plast. Reconstr. Surg. Glob. Open* **2013**, *1*, 1–2. [CrossRef]
91. Breuing, K.H.; Colwell, A.S. Inferolateral AlloDerm hammock for implant coverage in breast reconstruction. *Ann. Plast. Surg.* **2013**, *59*, 250–255. [CrossRef]
92. D'Aniello, C.; Cuomo, R.; Grimaldi, L.; Brandi, C.; Sisti, A.; Tassinari, J.; Nisi, G. Superior Pedicle Mammaplasty without Parenchymal Incisions after Massive Weight Loss. *J. Investig. Surg.* **2017**, *30*, 410–420. [CrossRef]
93. Berna, G.; Cawthorn, S.J.; Papaccio, G.; Balestrieri, N. Evaluation of a novel breast reconstruction technique using the Braxon® acellular dermal matrix: A new muscle-sparing breast reconstruction. *ANZ J. Surg.* **2017**, *87*, 493–498. [CrossRef] [PubMed]
94. Wazir, U.; Mokbel, K. The evolving role of pre-pectoral ADM-assisted implant-based immediate breast reconstruction following skin-sparing mastectomy. *Am. J. Surg.* **2018**, *216*, 639–640. [CrossRef] [PubMed]
95. Vidya, R.; Masia, J.; Cawthorn, S.; Berna, G.; Bozza, F.; Gardetto, A.; Kolacinska, A.; Dell'Antonia, F.; Tiengo, C.; Bassetto, F.; et al. Evaluation of the effectiveness of the prepectoral breast reconstruction with Braxon dermal matrix: First multicenter European report on 100 cases. *Breast J.* **2017**, *23*, 670–676. [CrossRef]
96. Kuwahara, M.; Hatoko, M.; Tada, H.; Tanaka, A.; Yurugi, S.; Mashiba, K. Distortion and movement of the expander during skin expansion. *Scand. J. Plast. Reconstr. Surg. Hand Surg.* **2003**, *37*, 22–27. [CrossRef]
97. Cheng, H.M.; McMillan, C.; Lipa, J.E.; Snell, L. A Qualitative Assessment of the Journey to Delayed Breast Reconstruction. *Plast. Surg.* **2017**, *25*, 157–162. [CrossRef]
98. Becker, H.; Lind, J.G., 2nd; Hopkins, E.G. Immediate Implant-based Prepectoral Breast Reconstruction Using a Vertical Incision. *Plast. Reconstr. Surg. Glob. Open* **2015**, *3*, e412. [CrossRef] [PubMed]
99. Baker, B.G.; Irri, R.; MacCallum, V.; Chattopadhyay, R.; Murphy, J.; Harvey, J.R. A Prospective Comparison of Short-Term Outcomes of Subpectoral and Prepectoral Strattice-Based Immediate Breast Reconstruction. *Plast. Reconstr. Surg.* **2018**, *141*, 1077–1084. [CrossRef]
100. Sigalove, S. Prepectoral breast reconstruction and radiotherapy—A closer look. *Gland Surg.* **2019**, *8*, 67–74. [CrossRef]
101. Walia, G.S.; Aston, J.; Bello, R.; Mackert, G.A.; Pedreira, R.A.; Cho, B.H.; Carl, H.M.; Rada, E.M.; Rosson, G.D.; Sacks, J.M. Prepectoral Versus Subpectoral Tissue Expander Placement: A Clinical and Quality of Life Outcomes Study. *Plast. Reconstr. Surg. Glob. Open* **2018**, *6*, e1731. [CrossRef]
102. Fracol, M.; Qiu, C.S.; Feld, L.N.; Chiu, W.K.; Kim, J.Y.S. Myotomy-Capsulotomy with Intramuscular Fat Grafting: A Novel Technique for Secondary Treatment of Prepectoral Upper Pole Defects in Breast Reconstruction. *Aesthet. Surg. J. Am. Soc. Aesthet. Plast. Surg.* **2019**, *39*, 454–459. [CrossRef]
103. Cuomo, R.; Giardino, F.R.; Neri, A.; Nisi, G.; Brandi, C.; Zerini, I.; Han, J.; Grimaldi, L. Optimization of Prepectoral Breast Reconstruction. *Breast Care* **2020**. [CrossRef]
104. Pittman, T.A.; Abbate, O.A.; Economides, J.M. The P1 Method: Prepectoral Breast Reconstruction to Minimize the Palpable Implant Edge and Upper Pole Rippling. *Ann. Plast. Surg.* **2018**, *80*, 487–492. [CrossRef]
105. Tasoulis, M.K.; Teoh, V.; Khan, A.; Montgomery, C.; Mohammed, K.; Gui, G. Acellular dermal matrices as an adjunct to implant breast reconstruction: Analysis of outcomes and complications. *Eur. J. Surg. Oncol.* **2020**, *46*, 511–515. [CrossRef]
106. Lohmander, F.; Lagergren, J.; Roy, P.G.; Johansson, H.; Brandberg, Y.; Eriksen, C.; Frisell, J. Implant Based Breast Reconstruction with Acellular Dermal Matrix: Safety Data from an Open-label, Multicenter, Randomized, Controlled Trial in the Setting of Breast Cancer Treatment. *Ann. Surg.* **2019**, *269*, 836–841. [CrossRef]
107. Antony, A.K.; McCarthy, C.M.; Cordeiro, P.G.; Mehrara, B.J.; Pusic, A.L.; Teo, E.H.; Arriaga, A.F.; Disa, J.J. Acellular human dermis implantation in 153 immediate two-stage tissue expander breast reconstructions: Determining the incidence and significant predictors of complications. *Plast. Reconstr. Surg.* **2010**, *125*, 1606–1614. [CrossRef]
108. Bernini, M.; Calabrese, C.; Cecconi, L.; Santi, C.; Gjondedaj, U.; Roselli, J.; Nori, J.; Fausto, A.; Orzalesi, L.; Casella, D. Subcutaneous Direct-to-Implant Breast Reconstruction: Surgical, Functional, and Aesthetic Results after Long-Term Follow-Up. *Plast. Reconstr. Surg. Glob. Open* **2015**, *3*, e574. [CrossRef]

109. Ibrahim, A.M.; Shuster, M.; Koolen, P.G.; Kim, K.; Taghinia, A.H.; Sinno, H.H.; Lee, B.T.; Lin, S.J. Analysis of the National Surgical Quality Improvement Program database in 19,100 patients undergoing implant-based breast reconstruction: Complication rates with acellular dermal matrix. *Plast. Reconstr. Surg.* **2013**, *132*, 1057–1066. [CrossRef]
110. Kamali, P.; Koolen, P.G.; Ibrahim, A.M.; Paul, M.A.; Dikmans, R.E.; Schermerhorn, M.L.; Lee, B.T.; Lin, S.J. Analyzing Regional Differences over a 15-Year Trend of One-Stage versus Two-Stage Breast Reconstruction in 941,191 Postmastectomy Patients. *Plast. Reconstr. Surg.* **2016**, *138*, 1e–14e. [CrossRef]
111. Abedi, N.; Ho, A.L.; Knox, A.; Tashakkor, Y.; Omeis, T.; Van Laeken, N.; Lennox, P.; Macadam, S.A. Predictors of Mastectomy Flap Necrosis in Patients Undergoing Immediate Breast Reconstruction: A Review of 718 Patients. *Ann. Plast. Surg.* **2016**, *76*, 629–634. [CrossRef]
112. Rubino, C.; Brongo, S.; Pagliara, D.; Cuomo, R.; Abbinante, G.; Campitiello, N.; Santanelli, F.; Chessa, D. Infections in breast implants: A review with a focus on developing countries. *J. Infect. Dev. Ctries* **2014**, *8*, 1089–1095. [CrossRef]
113. Powell-Brett, S.; Goh, S. Clinical and patient reported outcomes in breast reconstruction using acellular dermal matrix. *JPRAS Open* **2018**, *17*, 31–38. [CrossRef]
114. Bindingnavele, V.; Gaon, M.; Ota, K.S.; Kulber, D.A.; Lee, D.J. Use of acellular cadaveric dermis and tissue expansion in postmastectomy breast reconstruction. *J. Plast. Reconstr. Aesthet. Surg.* **2007**, *60*, 1214–1218. [CrossRef]
115. Disa, J.J.; Ad-El, D.D.; Cohen, S.M.; Cordeiro, P.G.; Hidalgo, D.A. The premature removal of tissue expanders in breast reconstruction. *Plast. Reconstr. Surg.* **1999**, *104*, 1662–1665. [CrossRef]
116. Munabi, N.C.; Olorunnipa, O.B.; Goltsman, D.; Rohde, C.H.; Ascherman, J.A. The ability of intra-operative perfusion mapping with laser-assisted indocyanine green angiography to predict mastectomy flap necrosis in breast reconstruction: A prospective trial. *J. Plast. Reconstr. Aesthet. Surg.* **2014**, *67*, 449–455. [CrossRef]
117. Apte, A.; Walsh, M.; Balaji, P.; Khor, B.; Chandrasekharan, S.; Chakravorty, A. Single stage immediate breast reconstruction with acellular dermal matrix and implant: Defining the risks and outcomes of post-mastectomy radiotherapy. *Surgeon* **2019**. [CrossRef]
118. Apte, A.; Walsh, M.; Chandrasekharan, S.; Chakravorty, A. Single-stage immediate breast reconstruction with acellular dermal matrix: Experience gained and lessons learnt from patient reported outcome measures. *Eur. J. Surg. Oncol.* **2016**, *42*, 39–44. [CrossRef]
119. Endara, M.; Chen, D.; Verma, K.; Nahabedian, M.Y.; Spear, S.L. Breast reconstruction following nipple-sparing mastectomy: A systematic review of the literature with pooled analysis. *Plast. Reconstr. Surg.* **2013**, *132*, 1043–1054. [CrossRef]
120. Hammond, D.C.; Schmitt, W.P.; O'Connor, E.A. Treatment of breast animation deformity in implant-based reconstruction with pocket change to the subcutaneous position. *Plast. Reconstr. Surg.* **2015**, *135*, 1540–1544. [CrossRef]
121. Pittman, T.A.; Fan, K.L.; Knapp, A.; Frantz, S.; Spear, S.L. Comparison of Different Acellular Dermal Matrices in Breast Reconstruction: The 50/50 Study. *Plast. Reconstr. Surg.* **2017**, *139*, 521–528. [CrossRef]
122. Spear, S.L.; Masden, D.; Rao, S.S.; Nahabedian, M.Y. Long-term outcomes of failed prosthetic breast reconstruction. *Ann. Plast. Surg.* **2013**, *71*, 286–291. [CrossRef]
123. Spear, S.L.; Schwartz, J.; Dayan, J.H.; Clemens, M.W. Outcome assessment of breast distortion following submuscular breast augmentation. *Aesthet. Plast. Surg.* **2009**, *33*, 44–48. [CrossRef]
124. Spear, S.L.; Sher, S.R.; Al-Attar, A.; Pittman, T. Applications of acellular dermal matrix in revision breast reconstruction surgery. *Plast. Reconstr. Surg.* **2014**, *133*, 1–10. [CrossRef]
125. Nelson, J.A.; Sobti, N.; Patel, A.; Matros, E.; McCarthy, C.M.; Dayan, J.H.; Disa, J.J.; Cordeiro, P.G.; Mehrara, B.J.; Pusic, A.L.; et al. The Impact of Obesity on Patient-Reported Outcomes Following Autologous Breast Reconstruction. *Ann. Surg. Oncol.* **2019**. [CrossRef]

126. Sadok, N.; Krabbe-Timmerman, I.S.; de Bock, G.H.; Werker, P.M.N.; Jansen, L. The Effect of Smoking and Body Mass Index on the Complication Rate of Alloplastic Breast Reconstruction. *Scand. J. Surg.* **2019**. [CrossRef]
127. Srinivasa, D.R.; Clemens, M.W.; Qi, J.; Hamill, J.B.; Kim, H.M.; Pusic, A.L.; Wilkins, E.G.; Butler, C.E.; Garvey, P.B. Obesity and Breast Reconstruction: Complications and Patient-Reported Outcomes in a Multicenter, Prospective Study. *Plast. Reconstr. Surg.* **2020**, *145*, 481e–490e. [CrossRef]

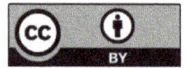

© 2020 by the author. Licensee MDPI, Basel, Switzerland. This article is an open access article distributed under the terms and conditions of the Creative Commons Attribution (CC BY) license (http://creativecommons.org/licenses/by/4.0/).

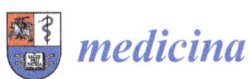

Review

Lipotransfer Strategies and Techniques to Achieve Successful Breast Reconstruction in the Radiated Breast

Kristina Crawford [1] and Matthew Endara [2,*]

1. Resident Physician, Vanderbilt University Medical Center, Nashville, TN 37232, USA; kristinaMcrawford@gmail.com
2. Plastic Surgeon, Maury Regional Medical Group, Columbia, TN 38401, USA
* Correspondence: matt.endara@gmail.com

Received: 27 August 2020; Accepted: 22 September 2020; Published: 1 October 2020

Abstract: Radiation therapy is frequently a critical component of breast cancer care but carries with it side effects that are particularly damaging to reconstructive efforts. Autologous lipotransfer has the ability to improve radiated skin throughout the body due to the pluripotent stem cells and multiple growth factors transferred therein. The oncologic safety of lipotransfer to the breasts is demonstrated in the literature and is frequently considered an adjunctive procedure for improving the aesthetic outcomes of breast reconstruction. Using lipotransfer as an integral rather than adjunctive step in the reconstructive process for breast cancer patients requiring radiation results in improved complication rates equivalent to those of nonradiated breasts, expanding options in these otherwise complicated cases. Herein, we provide a detailed review of the cellular toxicity conferred by radiotherapy and describe at length our approach to autologous lipotransfer in radiated breasts.

Keywords: lipotransfer; fat grafting; breast reconstruction; tissue expansion; radiotherapy; expander-to-implant; radiated breast

---

1. Introduction

Reconstruction of the breasts following the surgical management of cancer is associated with improved quality of life, feelings of well-being, and psychosocial development [1,2]. The objective of the reconstructive surgeon should be to offer options that facilitate these goals while minimizing potential complications. Between 2004 and 2015, 2.4 million women were diagnosed with breast cancer [3]. Partial mastectomy was the most frequent surgical treatment and implant reconstruction was the most common reconstructive choice [3]. Acellular dermal matrix (ADM) is utilized in approximately 50% of breast reconstructions [4].

Radiation in the patient's oncologic care is a well-known and well-studied risk factor for increased complications and reconstructive failure [5,6]. Since the appropriate management of cancer frequently requires radiation treatment (RT) to improve survival and recurrence rates, it is incumbent on the reconstructive surgeon to identify and implement strategies to compensate for this therapy. The traditional "gold standard" treatment for this has been the transfer of well-vascularized tissue in the form of a pedicled or free flap to reconstruct the resultant volume loss in the radiated breast. Though effective, these procedures may not always be available or the patient's preferred option. Lack of access to properly trained reconstructive microsurgeons, inexperienced hospitals, and a paucity of donor sites impact patients' ability to undergo these procedures. Patients may also wish to avoid procedures with potential donor site complications, increased operative time, requisite inpatient admission, or the longer postoperative recovery times that can be associated with these more complex surgeries. Autologous lipotransfer is a relatively simple procedure that is being increasingly recognized as a strategy in the radiated patient, with mounting evidence to support its use [7–15]. Though the ideal application of this technique remains debated in the literature, it is clearly becoming a critical and not simply adjunctive part of the reconstructive process in irradiated patients.

2. Use of Radiation in the Breast Cancer Patient

The use of RT in breast cancer patients irrefutably improves the survival and recurrence rates in lumpectomy and properly selected mastectomy patients [16–19]. Breast conserving therapy (BCT) as a treatment modality uses RT as a necessary step. As such, the vast majority of these patients are subject to RT as part of their treatment. The indications for use in mastectomy patients are expanding as well, with some centers offering it to as much as 70% of patients [19]. Indeed, a meta-analysis by the Early Breast Cancer Trialists Collaborative Group (EBCTCG) found improved rates for the 10-year recurrence and 20-year mortality in doing so [17]. The number of patients who require reconstruction and have been or will be exposed to RT is, therefore, increasing.

Irradiated tissues are associated with increased rates of surgical complication throughout the body [20,21]. This is especially true with radiated breast reconstruction, as evidenced by the higher rates of infection, capsular contracture, implant exposure, and overall reconstructive failure [22–38]. Though still the most common form of reconstruction being performed today, staged expander-to-implant-based reconstruction is especially sensitive to the unintended side effects of radiation. Interestingly, the timing of post-mastectomy radiotherapy may have a bearing on the complication rates [30,38]. Given the higher complication rate incurred by radiotherapy, some surgeons refuse to even offer an implant-based procedure to women who require radiation. Patients desiring procedures to correct asymmetries, ptosis, or macromastia following BCT can be at increased risk of complications such as delayed healing, prolonged edema, and breast loss necessitating flap reconstruction. Despite complications, these procedures are believed to be safe but with careful patient selection. One study found a pooled complication rate of 50% with mastopexy or a reduction in patients who had undergone BCT with RT [37]. Ultimately, an understanding of the harmful effect that radiation introduces to the surrounding tissues is paramount to success when designing treatment strategies for reconstruction in these patients.

The mechanisms by which RT is so effective at shrinking tumor size and local recurrence are the same ones that cause collateral side effects to local tissues. Radiation-induced tissue damage and the ensuing cellular and molecular response have been well-described in the literature [39–44]. The process occurs in three general phases: acute, latent, and late. The acute phase is thought to last from 0 to 6 months after exposure to radiation. This phase is characterized by damage to highly replicative cell lines through the initiation of cytokine cascades, the creation of reactive oxygen species, and the release of free radicals within the exposed cells. This property of RT is useful for causing apoptosis in cancer cells but is equally harmful to other proliferative cell lines such as basal keratinocytes and hair follicle stem cells. Damage to these regenerative cell lines results in the impairment of self-renewing abilities within the skin. Fibroblasts, endothelial cells, and epidermal cells within the radiation field are also affected, resulting in the release of a variety of molecular signals. This leads to the activation of the coagulation cascade, as well as increased inflammation, tissue remodeling, and epithelial regeneration. Finally, blood vessels, especially smaller arterioles and capillaries, are affected during this phase. These vessels demonstrate increased permeability and thus tissue edema, as well as the formation of fibrin plugs, with the resultant creation of local areas of ischemia.

The tissues proceed from the acute phase to a short latent period that is, as of yet, undefined but is believed to begin approximately 6 months after treatment [45,46]. The late-phase reactions occur next and can progress up to and beyond 20 years after initial exposure. The continued release of cytokines and growth factors results in prolonged fibroblast proliferation and progressive extracellular matrix deposition. Tissues become fibrotic, with a decrease in vascular density. These factors lead to sites inhospitable to surgical interventions, as they are stiff and have inadequate perfusion for healing. As such, these patients are frequently considered poor candidates for additional reconstructive procedures. Several studies have identified expander-to-implant surgeries as being particularly susceptible to these negative effects [23,25]. Patients desiring some form of breast reshaping after breast conservation therapy are equally approached with caution.

Strategies that take into account these harmful effects of radiation have been met with some success [47–52]. This includes delaying the expander-to-implant exchange procedure for 6 months to allow for the completion of the acute phase; using a counter incision in the IMF, thereby avoiding the more heavily radiated mastectomy incision line; and the use of autologous lipotransfer to physiologically reverse the harmful effects.

3. Autologous Lipotransfer to Regenerate Radiated Tissues

Though used for over 100 years to increase tissue bulk for cosmetic effect throughout the body, autologous lipotransfer is now seen as a particularly useful technique for treating radiodermatitis [53]. The reason it is so effective in this regard appears to be due to the multipotent adipose-derived stem cells, the adipose-derived regenerative cells transferred, and miscellaneous components of the stromal vascular fraction of the graft. It has been observed that adipose-derived stem cells (ASC) have the ability to regenerate new adipose tissue, ductal epithelium, and even nipple structures [54]. The mechanism by which adipose stem cells are capable of reversing the harmful effects of radiation is an area of active research [55]. It does appear that within radiated tissue the ASC is important, as it is capable of thriving and even proliferating in that ischemic environment [54]. Suspected mechanisms by which ASCs to promote the reversal of radiodermatitis are their ability to differentiate into lost cell types and to release paracrine signals with proangiogenic and anti-fibrotic effects.

Another factor that may contribute to the proangiogenic effect seen with lipotransfer into irradiated tissues is the inclusion of additional vessel-forming elements [56]. These include endothelial cells, pericytes, smooth muscle cells, and their progenitors capable of forming vascular cells and blood vessels. Experimental models transferring human fat to irradiated murine tissue has supported these findings. Indeed, the grafted tissue was found to have a decreased dermal thickness, reduction in collagen content, increase in vascular density, and overall improved fat graft retention.

Clinically, the beneficial effect of fat grafting in radiated patients has been demonstrated in several studies [8–10]. This technique for ameliorating the radiodermatitis of the breast is changing the way that reconstructive surgeons are approaching breast cancer patients. Initial concern over the potential for cancer activation limited the use of autologous lipotransfer in the breast. Multiple clinical studies, meta-analysis, and systematic reviews have failed to provide evidence to support this concern. Consequently, lipofilling had been used with increasing popularity in breast reconstruction, but typically as an adjunctive step to improve the final cosmetic result [57]. While oily cyst formation is a notable complication in a minority of patients, lipotransfer to the breast is generally regarded as a safe and well-tolerated procedure [58,59]. Moreover, the increased recognition of the positive effects on radiation tissue has resulted in the development of treatment protocols that incorporate it as an integral part of reconstructing these radiated patients.

4. Use of Autologous Lipotransfer in the Reconstruction of the Radiated Breast

Initial experience with lipotransfer in the radiated breast focused on using it to revive and prime post mastectomy skin flaps either after the completion of reconstruction or prior to attempting it [8,13–15]. These strategies were important for demonstrating efficacy in improving complication and failure rates but were limited in the cosmetic results they were able to obtain, delaying the overall time course.

Building on this, Ribuffo et al. presented 32 patients who underwent modified radical mastectomy followed by RT [7]. The patients were reconstructed in an immediate fashion at the time of mastectomy with the placement of tissue expanders in a submuscular plane. Half of the patients underwent between 1 and 2 separate autologous lipotransfer procedures as early as 6 weeks after the completion of radiotherapy before expander to implant exchange. They reported a 0% complication rate in their treatment arm and a 43% rate in the control group. Introducing lipotransfer as a separate but necessary part of their protocol was unique, and it became a formal part of their protocol for success.

Work by Serra-Renom et al. confirmed the utility of lipotransfer in 65 of their mastectomized irradiated patients by incorporating serial fat grafting into their protocol [9]. These patients underwent multiple fat grafting procedures, including before and at the time of expander to implant exchange. They found excellent clinical results with their technique. This study was limited, as the patients were not demonstrating significant acute effects of radiation in the form of radiodermatitis, and thus the severity of damage to the tissues was in question.

Our 3-stage lipo-approach to mastectomized irradiated patients is modeled on these previous studies and additional best available evidence for mitigating radiotoxicity (see Scheme 1). The hallmarks of our algorithm include the use of an ADM, maintenance of the expander in a fully inflated position during radiation, the delay of the expander-to-implant procedure for at least 6 months after radiotherapy completion, the use of a counter-incision at the inframammary fold (IMF) in cases of skin-sparing mastectomy (SSM), and the performance of a separate surgery whereby autologous fat is transferred to the radiated breast prior to the final exchange. Our algorithm is illustrated in Scheme 1. Comparing radiated breasts to our general non-radiated population as well as within for patients who had a bilateral mastectomy, whereby one breast was radiated and one was non-radiated, revealed equivalent complication rates ($p = 0.387$ and $p = 1$ respectively). Table 1 outlines our patient demographics. The clinical outcomes are detailed in Tables 2 and 3.

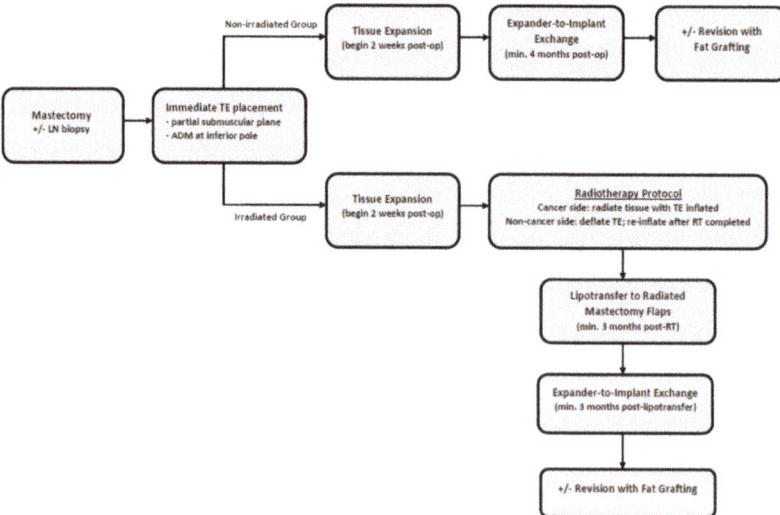

Scheme 1. Treatment algorithm. LN = lymph node; TE = Tissue Expander; ADM = acellular dermal matrix; RT = radiation treatment.

Table 1. Patient demographics and risk factors.

	Total No. of Patients (n = 131)	Non-Irradiated (n = 113; 86.26%)	Irradiated [1] (n = 18; 13.74%)	p-Value [2]
Categorical Variables		N (%)		
SSM	114 (87.02)	98 (86.73)	16 (88.89)	1
NSM	17 (12.98)	15 (13.27)	2 (11.11)	1
Smoking	21 (16.03)	17 (15.04)	4 (22.22)	0.489
Continuous Variables		Mean (SD)		p-Value [3]
Age		48.85 (10.35)	52.22 (9.51)	0.182
BMI		27.18 (7.27)	27.84 (6.47)	0.696

[1] External beam radiation; doses ranged from 4600 cGy to 5040 cGy. [2] Categorical p-values were derived using Fisher's exact test; [3] continuous p-values were derived using un-paired t-tests. SSM = Skin Sparing Mastectomy; NSM = Nipple Sparing Mastectomy; BMI = Body Mass Index.

Table 2. Patient outcomes.

	Total No. of Patients (n = 131)	Non-Irradiated (n = 113; 86.26%)	Irradiated (n = 18; 13.74%)	p-Value [1]
Categorical Variables		N (%)		
Complications (any)	13 (9.92)	10 (8.84)	3 (16.67)	0.387
Infection	2 (1.53)	2 (1.77)	0 (0)	1
Dehiscence	5 (3.82)	3 (2.65)	2 (11.11)	0.139
Reoperation	11 (8.39)	8 (7.08)	3 (16.67)	0.177
Implant Failure	4 (3.05)	3 (2.65)	1 (5.56)	0.451
Capsular Contracture	4 (3.05)	3 (2.65)	1 (5.56)	0.451

[1] Categorical p-values were derived using Fisher's exact test.

Table 3. Patient outcomes of internal controls [1].

	Total No. of Patients (n = 30)	Non-Irradiated (n = 15; 50%)	Irradiated (n = 15; 50%)	p-Value [2]
Categorical Variables		N (%)		
Complications (any)	5 (16.67)	2 (13.33)	3 (20)	1
Infection	0 (0)	0 (0)	0 (0)	-
Dehiscence	3 (10)	1 (6.67)	2 (13.33)	-
Reoperation	5 (16.67)	2 (13.33)	3 (20)	-
Implant Failure	1 (3.33)	0 (0)	1 (6.67)	-
Capsular Contracture	2 (6.67)	1 (6.67)	1 (6.67)	-

[1] Internal controls were patients who had one radiated and one non-radiated breast. [2] Categorical p-values were derived using Fisher's exact test.

A subset of patients who have undergone breast conservation therapy with lumpectomy followed by radiation desire either mastopexy or reduction to improve their postoperative appearance as well as improve the symmetry between their treated and untreated breast. The current recommendations are to limit offering these surgeries to carefully selected patients as long after radiation as possible. The use of fat grafting to "prime" the skin envelope as a separate procedure prior to attempting a reduction or a lift is an alternative strategy that has been successfully utilized in our practice (nonpublished) with reproducible and reliable results.

4.1. Three-Step Approach in the Mastectomy Patient Requiring Post Mastectomy Radiation

In radiation-naïve patients undergoing a mastectomy, the preoperative consultation includes a discussion of the three-stage approach to implant-based reconstruction, as well as the use of autologous flaps, should radiation be in question or required. Inherent in this approach is the use of flaps as a salvage procedure should implant failure arise. Patients who have already undergone radiation, such as previous breast conservation therapy patients now suffering a recurrence, are not candidates for this approach, and some form of autologous flap transfer is recommended.

Regardless of whether a patient would prefer flap or implant-based reconstruction, we prefer to proceed in a delayed immediate fashion. The placement of a tissue expander at the time of the mastectomy is therefore essential in this technique, precluding direct to implant or immediate flap reconstruction. Though evidence for the use of this technique applies to partial submuscular expander placement, it is currently being used for prepectoral reconstructions as well [60]. Cuomo et al. report better aesthetic results with prepectoral reconstruction [61]. In either case, the use of an acellular dermal matrix is considered an important part of the expander placement. The placement of this matrix creates a plane for ease of lipotransfer that is thought to be radioprotective.

The patient undergoes serial expansions starting two weeks after the index procedure. The breast to be radiated is expanded to the patient preference or the expander limit. On this side, we kept the tissue expander (TE) inflated during RT, as there is growing evidence that expander deflation leads to expander loss; skin dimpling; and the distortion of the inferior edge, leading to skin trauma upon re-inflation. [62,63]. An emerging study has also suggested decreased toxicity to the chest wall and underlying structures with the maintenance of TE inflation during RT [64]. In those who have undergone bilateral mastectomy, the non-radiated side is deflated prior to radiation, as this more effectively keeps this tissue out of the radiation field. The patient is monitored through their RT with a clinic visit at the halfway mark and following the completion of treatment. One week after the completion of radiation, the non-radiated breast is then easily re-inflated.

The patient is then subject to a 3-month waiting period prior to their next procedure: autologous lipotransfer to the radiated breast. At this point, the patient is taken back to the operating room for whole-breast fat grafting. This procedure is performed by utilizing a superwet technique for liposuction into a revolve fat transfer harvest system. Prior to the injection of the fat, pre-tunneling is performed within the subcutaneous space. The correct space is identified under direct visualization through a 1 cm incision within the mastectomy scar. The avoidance of using sharp tipped instruments is important during this step to avoid rupturing the expander. Scar tissue bands that may block the ability to uniformly inject the fat are severed using a riveted fat harvest cannula with a saw-type motion. The expander is then deflated by 60–100 mL to make room for the transfer of the fat. It is important to avoid over deflation, as the fat still requires a flat plane to be placed in a string of pearls fashion.

The fat is then processed with three washes of warm lactated ringers. It is transferred from the revolve to a 60 mL syringe, then into 3 mL syringes for transfer. The majority of the fat is injected through the incision. If additional access sites are needed to optimize the angle of delivery, they can be made with a 16-gauge needle while tenting the skin from the inside with a fat-grafting cannula to protect the device. Constant motion of the syringe while injecting the fat is critical to avoid the clumping of the fat graft and subsequent poor take. Enough fat is injected to fill the space by injecting at least as much as the fluid removed, but not to the point of skin discoloration or the creation of an overly taut skin envelope.

Following the completion of this step, the patient is monitored closely with weekly follow-up visits for the 3 weeks after surgery. If additional expansion is desired, this can be attempted at 1-month post fat grating. The patient is subject to another 3-month waiting period before their final surgery. This is timed to optimize the chances that the lipoaspirate will positively affect the acute phase of radiation injury while performing the surgery during the latent phase.

The patient is taken back to the operating room once more for the removal of the expander and the placement of the final implant. In cases of skin-sparing mastectomy, a counter-incision is utilized within the inframammary fold. Patients who have undergone a nipple-sparing mastectomy using an IMF incision are accessed by extending the incision laterally. Any requisite capsular modifications are able to be performed at this time to not only enhance the final shape of the reconstructed breast but also address any contraction that had occurred as a result of radiation. The implant is introduced using a touch-free technique. Closure is performed in layers using a buried, monofilament dissolvable suture. Please see patient Figures 1–3.

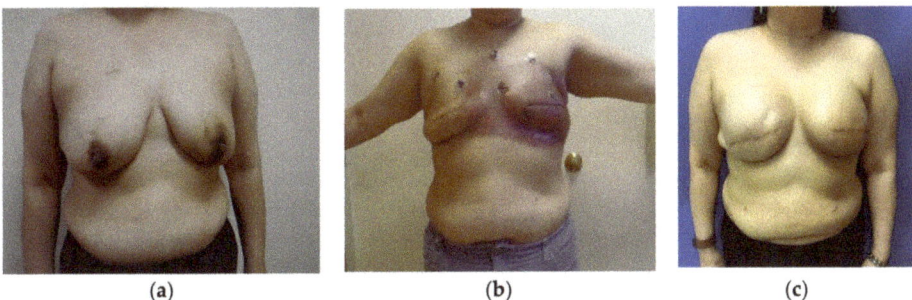

Figure 1. (**a**) Prior to bilateral mastectomy and 6 weeks after attempted lumpectomy with positive margins; (**b**) 10 weeks status-post bilateral mastectomy with immediate TE placement and halfway through radiotherapy regimen, with severe radiodermatitis; (**c**) 22 months following expander-to-implant exchange.

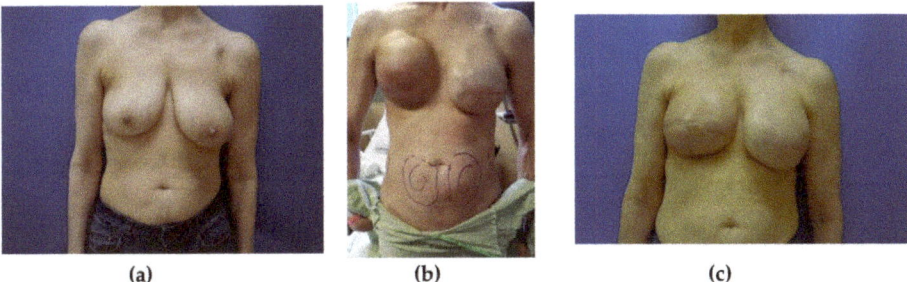

Figure 2. (**a**) Newly diagnosed right breast cancer prior to bilateral mastectomy; (**b**) five months after bilateral mastectomy with immediate TE placement and three months after radiotherapy completion, photo taken on the day of lipotransfer surgery with markings for fat harvest from abdomen; (**c**) seven months following lipotransfer to right breast and four months post expander-to-implant exchange.

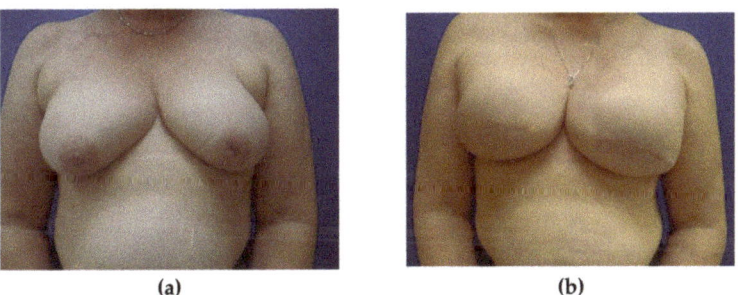

Figure 3. (**a**) Newly diagnosed left breast cancer prior to bilateral mastectomy; (**b**) six months after the completion of expander-to-implant reconstruction, near normal skin coloration and character noted. Patient previously underwent radiation of the left breast, followed three months later by lipotransfer to irradiated side, and expander-to-implant exchange performed after three additional months.

4.2. Two-Stage Approach to BCT Patients Desiring Oncoplastic Mastopexy or Reduction After Completion of RT

Eligible patients typically present with severe asymmetry following the completion of their breast conservation therapy combined with ptosis and/or macromastia. These patients are counseled on the risks of operating in a previously radiated surgical field and the benefit of priming the tissues with autologous lipotransfer before doing so. A two-step approach is offered, with the first procedure consisting of a lift/reduction of the nonradiated breast and fat grafting to the radiated breast. The mastopexy/reduction of the radiated side is performed at least 3 months later.

The fat-grafting technique is similar as for mastectomy patients, with the preferred plane of injection remaining in the subcutaneous space. Care is taken not to inject directly into the breast tissue for multiple reasons. The subcutaneous plane is the target of transfer, as we are trying to reverse the negative radiation effects on those regenerative cell lines that, if damaged, will lead to increased risk in the final breast shaping procedure. Injection into the breast tissue would not accomplish this goal and, though not proven by data, would be more concerning from an oncologic perspective. Multiple patients have been operated on in this manner by the primary author, with the largest complication being persistent asymmetry that was still improved from before surgery. The technique has allowed for a reduction in the selectivity for offering breast reshaping in previously radiated fields, as has been recommended by previous authors.

5. Conclusions

The recognition of the regenerative properties of lipoaspirate in radiated fields is leading to the simplification of breast reconstruction in this otherwise complicated patient population. The optimal strategy for this requires knowledge of the harmful effects of radiation, their time course, and the biomolecular pathways by which lipoaspirate reverses them. Though not yet fully understood, it is clear that applying autologous lipotransfer can significantly improve breast reconstruction outcomes in irradiated patients. The ease of these fat-grafting procedures along with their use and application throughout the body makes them very well-known to most plastic surgeons and may be leading to a paradigm shift in approaching the radiated breast. This has the potential to improve options and access to reconstruction for this ever-growing patient group.

Author Contributions: Conceptualization, methodology, and writing, M.E. Writing, edits, tables, K.C. All authors have read and agreed to the published version of the manuscript.

Funding: This research received no external funding.

Conflicts of Interest: The authors declare no conflict of interest. No authors have any relevant financial disclosures related to the research performed and presented. None of the authors have a financial interest in any of the products, devices, or drugs mentioned in this manuscript. No additional sources of funding were used or received to support the work presented in this article.

References

1. Fanakidou, I.; Zyga, S.; Alikari, V.; Tsironi, M.; Stathoulis, J.; Theofilou, P. Mental health, loneliness, and illness perception outcomes in quality of life among young breast cancer patients after mastectomy: The role of breast reconstruction. *Qual. Life Res.* **2018**, *27*, 539–543. [CrossRef] [PubMed]
2. Sisco, M.; Johnson, D.B.; Wang, C.; Rasinski, K.; Rundell, V.L.; Yao, K.A. The quality-of-life benefits of breast reconstruction do not diminish with age. *J. Surg. Oncol.* **2015**, *111*, 663–668. [CrossRef] [PubMed]
3. Sisti, A.; Huayllani, M.T.; Boczar, D.; Restrepo, D.J.; Spaulding, A.C.; Emmanuel, G.; Bagaria, S.P.; McLaughlin, S.; Parker, A.S.; Forte, A.J. Breast cancer in women: A descriptive analysis of the national cancer database. *Acta Biomed.* **2020**, *91*, 332–341. [CrossRef] [PubMed]
4. Cuomo, R. Submuscular and pre-pectoral ADM assisted immediate breast reconstruction: A literature review. *Medicina* **2020**, *56*, 256. [CrossRef] [PubMed]
5. Mericli, A.F.; Sharabi, S.E. Breast implants and radiation. *Semin. Plast. Surg.* **2019**, *33*, 240–246. [CrossRef]

6. See, M.S.F.; Farhadi, J. Radiation therapy and immediate breast reconstruction: Novel approaches and evidence base for radiation effects on the reconstructed breast. *Clin. Plast. Surg.* **2018**, *45*, 13–24. [CrossRef]
7. Ribuffo, D.; Atzeni, M.; Guerra, M.; Bucher, S.; Politi, C.; Deidda, M.; Atzori, F.; Dessì, M.; Madeddu, C.; Lay, G. Treatment of irradiated expanders: Protective lipofilling allows immediate prosthetic breast reconstruction in the setting of postoperative radiotherapy. *Aesthet. Plast. Surg.* **2013**, *37*, 1146–1152. [CrossRef]
8. Rigotti, G.; Marchi, A.; Galiè, M.; Baroni, G.; Benati, D.; Krampera, M.; Pasini, A.; Sbarbati, A. Clinical treatment of radiotherapy tissue damage by lipoaspirate transplant: A healing process mediated by adipose-derived adult stem cells. *Plast. Reconstr. Surg.* **2007**, *119*, 1409–1422. [CrossRef]
9. Serra-Renom, J.M.; Muñoz-Olmo, J.L.; Serra-Mestre, J.M. Fat grafting in postmastectomy breast reconstruction with expanders and prostheses in patients who have received radiotherapy: Formation of new subcutaneous tissue. *Plast. Reconstr. Surg.* **2010**, *125*, 12–18. [CrossRef]
10. Jackson, I.T.; Simman, R.; Tholen, R.; di Nick, V.D. A successful long-term method of fat grafting: Recontouring of a large subcutaneous postradiation thigh defect with autologous fat transplantation. *Aesthet. Plast. Surg.* **2001**, *25*, 165–169. [CrossRef]
11. Kim, S.S.; Kawamoto, H.K.; Kohan, E.; Bradley, J.P. Reconstruction of the irradiated orbit with autogenous fat grafting for improved ocular implant. *Plast. Reconstr. Surg.* **2010**, *126*, 213–220. [CrossRef] [PubMed]
12. Phulpin, B.; Gangloff, P.; Tran, N.; Bravetti, P.; Merlin, J.L.; Dolivet, G. Rehabilitation of irradiated head and neck tissues by autologous fat transplantation. *Plast. Reconstr. Surg.* **2009**, *123*, 1187–1197. [CrossRef] [PubMed]
13. Missana, M.C.; Laurent, I.; Barreau, L.; Balleyguier, C. Autologous fat transfer in reconstructive breast surgery: Indications, technique and results. *Eur. J. Surg. Oncol.* **2007**, *33*, 685–690. [CrossRef] [PubMed]
14. Panettiere, P.; Marchetti, L.; Accorsi, D. The serial free fat transfer in irradiated prosthetic breast reconstructions. *Aesthet. Plast. Surg.* **2009**, *33*, 695–700. [CrossRef]
15. Salgarello, M.; Visconti, G.; Barone-Adesi, L. Fat grafting and breast reconstruction with implant: Another option for irradiated breast cancer patients. *Plast. Reconstr. Surg.* **2012**, *129*, 317–329. [CrossRef]
16. Clarke, M.; Collins, R.; Darby, S.; Davies, C.; Elphinstone, P.; Evans, V.M.; Godwin, J.; Gray, R.; Hicks, C.; James, S.; et al. Effects of radiotherapy and of differences in the extent of surgery for early breast cancer on local recurrence and 15-year survival: An overview of the randomised trials. *Lancet* **2005**, *366*, 2087–2106.
17. McGale, P.; Taylor, C.; Correa, C.; Cutter, D.; Duane, F.; Ewertz, M.; Gray, R.; Mannu, G.; Peto, R.; Whelan, T.; et al. Effect of radiotherapy after mastectomy and axillary surgery on 10-year recurrence and 20-year breast cancer mortality: Meta-analysis of individual patient data for 8135 women in 22 randomised trials. *Lancet* **2014**, *383*, 2127–2135.
18. American Cancer Society. *Breast Cancer Facts & Figures 2017–2018*; American Cancer Society: Atlanta, GA, USA, 2018.
19. Delaney, G.; Barton, M.; Jacob, S. Estimation of an optimal radiotherapy utilization rate for breast carcinoma: A review of the evidence. *Cancer* **2003**, *98*, 1977–1986. [CrossRef]
20. Robinson, D.W. The hazards of surgery in irradiated tissue. *AMA Arch. Surg.* **1955**, *71*, 410–418. [CrossRef]
21. Robinson, D.W. Surgical problems in the excision and repair of radiated tissue. *Plast. Reconstr. Surg.* **1975**, *55*, 41–49. [CrossRef]
22. Rudolph, R. Complications of surgery for radiotherapy skin damage. *Plast. Reconstr. Surg.* **1982**, *70*, 179–185. [CrossRef] [PubMed]
23. Cordeiro, P.G.; Pusic, A.L.; Disa, J.J.; McCormick, B.; van Zee, K. Irradiation after immediate tissue expander/implant breast reconstruction: Outcomes, complications, aesthetic results, and satisfaction among 156 patients. *Plast. Reconstr. Surg.* **2004**, *113*, 877–881. [CrossRef] [PubMed]
24. Jhaveri, J.D.; Rush, S.C.; Kostroff, K.; DeRisi, D.; Farber, L.A.; Maurer, V.E.; Bosworth, J.L. Clinical outcomes of postmastectomy radiation therapy after immediate breast reconstruction. *Int. J. Radiat. Oncol. Biol. Phys.* **2008**, *72*, 859–865. [CrossRef]
25. Tallet, A.V.; Salem, N.; Moutardier, V.; Ananian, P.; Braud, A.-C.; Zalta, R.; Cowen, D.; Houvenaeghel, G. Radiotherapy and immediate two-stage breast reconstruction with a tissue expander and implant: Complications and esthetic results. *Int. J. Radiat. Oncol. Biol. Phys.* **2003**, *57*, 136–142. [CrossRef]
26. Krueger, E.A.; Wilkins, E.G.; Strawderman, M.; Cederna, P.; Goldfarb, S.; A Vicini, F.; Pierce, L.J. Complications and patient satisfaction following expander/implant breast reconstruction with and without radiotherapy. *Int. J. Radiat. Oncol. Biol. Phys.* **2001**, *49*, 713–721. [CrossRef]

27. Kronowitz, S.J.; Hunt, K.K.; Kuerer, H.M.; Babiera, G.; McNeese, M.D.; Buchholz, T.A.; Strom, E.A.; Robb, G.L. Delayed-immediate breast reconstruction. *Plast. Reconstr. Surg.* **2004**, *113*, 1617–1628. [CrossRef] [PubMed]
28. Spear, S.L.; Majidian, A. Immediate breast reconstruction in two stages using textured, integrated-valve tissue expanders and breast implants: A retrospective review of 171 consecutive breast reconstructions from 1989 to 1996. *Plast. Reconstr. Surg.* **1998**, *101*, 53–63. [CrossRef] [PubMed]
29. Alderman, A.K.; Wilkins, E.G.; Kim, H.M.; Lowery, J.C. Complications in postmastectomy breast reconstruction: Two-year results of the Michigan Breast Reconstruction Outcome Study. *Plast. Reconstr. Surg.* **2002**, *109*, 2265–2274. [CrossRef]
30. Ricci, J.A.; Epstein, S.; Momoh, A.O.; Lin, S.J.; Singhal, D.; Lee, B.T. A meta-analysis of implant-based breast reconstruction and timing of adjuvant radiation therapy. *J. Surg. Res.* **2017**, *218*, 108–116. [CrossRef]
31. Ascherman, J.A.; Hanasono, M.M.; Newman, M.I.; Hughes, D.B. Implant reconstruction in breast cancer patients treated with radiation therapy. *Plast. Reconstr. Surg.* **2006**, *117*, 359–365. [CrossRef]
32. Anker, C.J.; Hymas, R.V.; Ahluwalia, R.; Kokeny, K.E.; Avizonis, V.; Boucher, K.M.; Neumayer, L.A.; Agarwal, J.P. The effect of radiation on complication rates and patient satisfaction in breast reconstruction using temporary tissue expanders and permanent implants. *Breast J.* **2015**, *21*, 233–240. [CrossRef] [PubMed]
33. Sullivan, S.R.; Fletcher, D.R.; Isom, C.D.; Isik, F.F. True incidence of all complications following immediate and delayed breast reconstruction. *Plast. Reconstr. Surg.* **2008**, *122*, 19–28. [CrossRef] [PubMed]
34. Poppe, M.M.; Agarwal, J.P. Breast reconstruction with postmastectomy radiation: Choices and tradeoffs. *J. Clin. Oncol.* **2017**, *35*, 2467–2470. [CrossRef] [PubMed]
35. Jagsi, R.; Momoh, A.O.; Qi, J.; Hamill, J.B.; Billig, J.; Kim, H.M.; Pusic, A.L.; Wilkins, E.G. Impact of radiotherapy on complications and patient-reported outcomes after breast reconstruction. *J. Natl. Cancer. Inst.* **2018**, *110*, 157–165. [CrossRef]
36. Barnea, Y.; Bracha, G.; Arad, E.; Gur, E.; Inbal, A. Breast reduction and mastopexy for repair of asymmetry after breast conservation therapy: Lessons learned. *Aesthet. Plast. Surg.* **2019**, *43*, 600–607. [CrossRef]
37. Spear, S.L.; Rao, S.S.; Patel, K.M.; Nahabedian, M.Y. Reduction mammaplasty and mastopexy in previously irradiated breasts. *Aesthet. Surg. J.* **2014**, *34*, 74–78. [CrossRef]
38. Oliver, J.D.; Boczar, D.; Huayllani, M.T.; Restrepo, D.J.; Sisti, A.; Manrique, O.J.; Broer, P.N.; McLaughlin, S.; Rinker, B.D.; Forte, A.J. Postmastectomy radiation therapy (PMRT) before and after 2-stage expander-implant breast reconstruction: A systematic review. *Medicina* **2019**, *55*, 226. [CrossRef]
39. Hymes, S.R.; Strom, E.A.; Fife, C. Radiation dermatitis: Clinical presentation, pathophysiology, and treatment 2006. *J. Am. Acad. Dermatol.* **2006**, *54*, 28–46. [CrossRef]
40. Hauer-Jensen, M.; Fink, L.M.; Wang, J. Radiation injury and the protein C pathway. *Crit. Care Med.* **2004**, *32*, S325–S330. [CrossRef]
41. López, E.; Guerrero, R.; Núñez, M.I.; Del Moral, R.; Villalobos, M.; Martínez-Galán, J.; Valenzuela, M.T.; Muñoz-Gámez, J.A.; Oliver, F.J.; Martín-Oliva, D.; et al. Early and late skin reactions to radiotherapy for breast cancer and their correlation with radiation-induced DNA damage in lymphocytes. *Breast Cancer Res.* **2005**, *7*, R690. [CrossRef]
42. Yarnold, J.; Brotons, M.C.V. Pathogenetic mechanisms in radiation fibrosis. *Radiother. Oncol.* **2010**, *97*, 149–161. [CrossRef] [PubMed]
43. Martin, M.; Lefaix, J.L.; Delanian, S. TGF-β1 and radiation fibrosis: A master switch and a specific therapeutic target? *Int. J. Radiat. Oncol. Biol. Phys.* **2000**, *47*, 277–290. [CrossRef]
44. Wei, J.; Wang, B.; Wang, H.; Meng, L.; Zhao, Q.; Li, X.; Xin, Y.; Jiang, X. Radiation-induced normal tissue damage: Oxidative stress and epigenetic mechanisms. *Oxid. Med. Cell. Longev.* **2019**, *2019*. [CrossRef] [PubMed]
45. Bentzen, S.M.; Thames, H.D.; Overgaard, M. Latent-time estimation for late cutaneous and subcutaneous radiation reactions in a single-follow-up clinical study. *Radiother. Oncol.* **1989**, *15*, 267–274. [CrossRef]
46. Arcangeli, G.; Friedman, M.; Paoluzi, R. A quantitative study of late radiation effect on normal skin and subcutaneous tissues in human beings. *Br. J. Radiol.* **1974**, *47*, 44–50. [CrossRef]
47. Nahabedian, M.Y. Minimizing incisional dehiscence following 2-stage prosthetic breast reconstruction in the setting of radiation therapy. *Gland Surg.* **2013**, *2*, 133.

48. Fowble, B.; Park, C.; Wang, F.; Peled, A.; Alvarado, M.; Ewing, C.; Esserman, L.; Foster, R.; Sbitany, H.; Hanlon, A. Rates of reconstruction failure in patients undergoing immediate reconstruction with tissue expanders and/or implants and postmastectomy radiation therapy. *Int. J. Radiat. Oncol. Biol. Phys.* **2015**, *92*, 634–641. [CrossRef]
49. Kronowitz, S.J. State of the art and science in postmastectomy breast reconstruction. *Plast. Reconstr. Surg.* **2015**, *135*, 755e–771e. [CrossRef]
50. Percec, I.; Bucky, L.P. Successful prosthetic breast reconstruction after radiation therapy. *Ann. Plast. Surg.* **2008**, *60*, 527–531. [CrossRef]
51. Kronowitz, S.J.; Robb, G.L. Radiation therapy and breast reconstruction: A critical review of the literature. *Plast. Reconstr. Surg.* **2009**, *124*, 395–408. [CrossRef]
52. Kronowitz, S.J. Current status of implant-based breast reconstruction in patients receiving postmastectomy radiation therapy. *Plast. Reconstr. Surg.* **2012**, *130*, 513e–523e. [CrossRef] [PubMed]
53. Borrelli, M.R.; Patel, R.A.; Sokol, J.; Nguyen, D.; Momeni, A.; Longaker, M.T.; Wan, D.C. Fat chance: The rejuvenation of irradiated skin. *Plast. Reconstr. Surg. Glob. Open* **2019**, *7*, e2092. [CrossRef] [PubMed]
54. Conci, C.; Bennati, L.; Bregoli, C.; Buccino, F.; Danielli, F.; Gallan, M.; Gjini, E.; Raimondi, M.T. Tissue engineering and regenerative medicine strategies for the female breast. *J. Tissue Eng. Regen. Med.* **2020**, *14*, 369–387. [CrossRef] [PubMed]
55. Kumar, R.; Griffin, M.; Adigbli, G.; Kalavrezos, N.; Butler, P.E. Lipotransfer for radiation-induced skin fibrosis. *Br. J. Surg.* **2016**, *103*, 950–961. [CrossRef]
56. Hong, K.Y.; Yim, S.; Kim, H.J.; Jin, U.S.; Lim, S.; Eo, S.R.; Chang, H.; Minn, K.W. The fate of the adipose-derived stromal cells during angiogenesis and adipogenesis after cell-assisted lipotransfer. *Plast. Reconstr. Surg.* **2018**, *141*, 365–375. [CrossRef]
57. Zheng, D.-N.; Li, Q.; Lei, H.; Zheng, S.-W.; Xie, Y.-Z.; Xu, Q.-H.; Yun, X.; Pu, L.L. Autologous fat grafting to the breast for cosmetic enhancement: Experience in 66 patients with long-term follow up. *J. Plast. Reconstr. Aesthet. Surg.* **2008**, *61*, 792–798. [CrossRef]
58. Tassinari, J.; Sisti, A.; Zerini, I.; Idone, F.; Nisi, G. Oil cysts after breast augmentation with autologous fat grafting. *Plast. Reconstr. Surg.* **2016**, *137*, 244e–245e. [CrossRef]
59. Kontoes, P.; Gounnaris, G. Complications of fat transfer for breast augmentation. *Aesthet. Plast. Surg.* **2017**, *41*, 1078–1082. [CrossRef]
60. Sbitany, H.; Piper, M.; Lentz, R. Prepectoral breast reconstruction: A safe alternative to submuscular prosthetic reconstruction following nipple-sparing mastectomy. *Plast. Reconstr. Surg.* **2017**, *140*, 432–443. [CrossRef]
61. Cuomo, R.; Giardino, F.R.; Neri, A.; Nisi, G.; Brandi, C.; Zerini, I.; Jingjian, H.; Grimaldi, L. Optimization of prepectoral breast reconstruction. *Breast Care* **2020**. [CrossRef]
62. Woo, K.J.; Paik, J.M.; Bang, S.I.; Mun, G.H.; Pyon, J.K. The impact of expander inflation/deflation status during adjuvant radiotherapy on the complications of immediate two-stage breast reconstruction. *Aesthet. Plast. Surg.* **2017**, *41*, 551–559. [CrossRef] [PubMed]
63. Ozden, B.C.; Guven, E.; Aslay, I.; Kemikler, G.; Olgac, V.; Soluk-Tekkesin, M.; Serarslan, B.; Ulug, B.T.; Bilgin-Karabulut, A.; Arinci, A.; et al. Does partial expander deflation exacerbate the adverse effects of radiotherapy in two-stage breast reconstruction? *World J. Surg. Oncol.* **2012**, *10*, 44. [CrossRef] [PubMed]
64. Amro, H.; Aydogan, B.; Perevalova, E.; Stepaniak, C.; Golden, D.; McCabe, B.; Endara, M.; McCall, A. Optimal tissue expander inflation volume for post-mastectomy radiotherapy. In Proceedings of the American Association of Physicists in Medicine Annual Meeting, Denver, CO, USA, 30 July–3 August 2017.

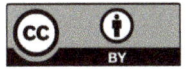

© 2020 by the authors. Licensee MDPI, Basel, Switzerland. This article is an open access article distributed under the terms and conditions of the Creative Commons Attribution (CC BY) license (http://creativecommons.org/licenses/by/4.0/).

Article

Protocol for Prevention and Monitoring of Surgical Site Infections in Implant-Based Breast Reconstruction: Preliminary Results

Giovanni Papa, Andrea Frasca *, Nadia Renzi, Chiara Stocco, Giuseppe Pizzolato, Vittorio Ramella and Zoran Marij Arnež

Plastic and Reconstructive Surgery Unit, Department of Medical, Surgical and Health Sciences, University of Trieste, 34100 Trieste, Italy; giovanni.papa@asugi.sanita.fvg.it (G.P.); nadia.renzi@asugi.sanita.fvg.it (N.R.); chiara.stocco@asugi.sanita.fvg.it (C.S.); giuseppe.pizzolato@asugi.sanita.fvg.it (G.P.); vittorio.ramella@asugi.sanita.fvg.it (V.R.); zoranmarij.arnez@asugi.sanita.fvg.it (Z.M.A.)
* Correspondence: andreafrasca.af@gmail.com

Abstract: Surgical site infection in implant-based breast reconstruction is a complication with variable incidence reported in the literature. Due to potential loss of implant and reconstruction, it can have a strong psychological impact on patients. *Background and objectives:* This study aimed primarily at analyzing the current status of the surgical site infection (SSI), (type, time of onset, clinical presentation, pathogens and management) in patients who underwent implant-based breast reconstruction at our Breast Unit. Secondarily, we wanted to establish whether introduction of a new, updated evidence-based protocol for infection prevention can reduce SSI in implant-based breast reconstruction. *Materials and Methods:* A single-center retrospective study was performed primarily to evaluate the incidence and features of SSI after implant-based breast reconstruction from 2007 to 2020. In June 2020, a protocol for prevention of SSI in implant-based breast reconstruction was introduced in clinical practice. Secondarily, a data analysis of all patients who underwent implant-based breast reconstruction in compliance with this protocol was performed after preliminarily assessing its efficacy. *Results:* 756 women were evaluated after mastectomy and implant-based breast reconstruction for breast cancer. A total of 26 surgical site infections were detected. The annual incidence of SSI decreased over time (range 0–11.76%). Data relating to infections' features, involved pathogens and implemented treatments were obtained. Since the introduction of the protocol, 22 patients have been evaluated, for a total of 29 implants. No early infections occurred. *Conclusions:* Surgical site infection rates at our Breast Unit are comparable to those reported in the literature. The SSI rates have shown a decreasing trend over the years. No SSI has occurred since the introduction of the prevention protocol for surgical site infection in June 2020.

Keywords: breast reconstruction; implant; infection; prevention; antibiotic prophylaxis; complication

1. Introduction

Surgical site infection (SSI) is one of the most common healthcare-associated infections (HAIs) and a major cause of increased hospital stay and mortality. SSI is a significant surgical complication in prosthetic breast reconstruction. The incidence reported in literature ranges from less than 1% up to 43% [1–4]. This variability can be explained by the absence of a unique definition, which could allow a diagnosis based on standardized criteria. According to the National Nosocomial Infection Surveillance System (NNIS), SSI is related to the surgical procedure and typically occurs within 30 days after surgery. In the case of implant-based breast reconstruction, this interval is prolonged to one year after surgery [5]. Three types of SSI are proposed by the Centers for Disease Control and Prevention (CDC): superficial incisional, deep incisional and organ and space SSI.

The clinical diagnosis of SSI is made by observing the classic signs of inflammation, (redness, delayed healing, fever, pain, tenderness, warmth, or swelling).

The risks for SSIs after the placement of prosthetic implants are multiple and have been extensively investigated [6–11]. They are related to the patient (age, smoking, obesity, diabetes mellitus, immunosuppression, presence of simultaneous infections or bacterial colonization, etc.) or to the surgical procedure (pre-operative shower and skin preparation, duration and repetition of hand washing, skin antisepsis, operative time, antibiotic prophylaxis, sterilization of surgical instruments, use of prosthetic material, drainage, intra-operative hypothermia, etc.)

SSI risk assessment is based on the National Healthcare Safety Network (NHSN) risk index [12], consisting of three equally weighted factors: the American Society of Anesthesiologists (ASA) score (3, 4, or 5), wound classification (contaminated or dirty), and operative time in minutes (>75th percentile). Each risk factor represents 1 point; thus, the NHSN SSI risk index ranges from 0 (lowest risk) to 3 (greatest risk).

The most frequently isolated pathogens in surgical site infections are *S. aureus* and Coagulase-negative staphylococci. However, the number of infectious complications due to multi-drug resistant (MDR) microorganisms is increasing, and the isolation of these pathogens in biological materials is associated with poor clinical outcomes. Among the multi-drug resistant (MDR) microorganisms, the most common ones include Methicillin-resistant *S. aureus* (MRSA), *Streptococcus*, and Gram-negative bacteria, such as *Pseudomonas* [13]. It has been shown that a large proportion of SSIs originate from the patients' own flora. Nasal carriage of *S. aureus* is now considered a well-defined risk factor for subsequent infection in various groups of patients [14,15]. Several interventional studies have attempted to reduce the infection rates by eradicating nasal carriage (screening for *S. aureus*, nasal decolonization by mupirocin, skin decontamination) [16,17].

In implant-based breast reconstruction, SSI could lead to prolonged hospitalization, re-intervention, multiple outpatient checks, or even to the loss of the reconstruction. Infections in prosthetic reconstruction correlate with the increased incidence of capsular contracture [18], one of the main indications for surgical revision.

No consensus exists regarding the duration of antibiotic prophylaxis and whether it should be continued after surgery in the presence of a drain close to the implant or in selected high-risk patients. A customized approach to this issue seems to be the most appropriate; in fact, some patients with certain risk factors such as diabetes mellitus, obesity, or low-quality mastectomy flaps can benefit from prolonged antibiotic administration [19].

The primary aim of our study is to analyze the current status of infection rates at our institution (type of infection, timing of onset, clinical manifestations, pathogens involved, and potential treatments) in patients undergoing prosthetic breast reconstruction. The secondary aim is to evaluate the effectiveness of a new Prevention Protocol for SSI by analyzing the patients' data.

2. Materials and Methods

2.1. Retrospective Analysis

We conducted a monocentric study at the Plastic and Reconstructive Surgery Unit of Azienda Sanitaria Universitaria Giuliano Isontina (ASUGI)—Trieste to retrospectively review SSIs' rates and characteristics among patients undergoing prosthetic breast reconstruction (immediate direct-to-implant and two-stage tissue expander/implant breast reconstruction) between January 2007 and June 2020.

The analyzed SSIs' characteristics include the type of diagnosed infection, the interval between surgery, the diagnosis of infection, the symptoms associated with infection, the pathogens isolated from microbial cultures, and the number of revision surgeries.

2.2. Prospective Analysis

We prospectively enroll all patients undergoing implant-based breast reconstruction from the introduction of our Prevention Protocol for SSIs (June 2020) in a prospective study aimed at evaluation of its effectiveness.

Prevention Protocol for SSIs involves a pre-operative phase, reported in Box 1, concerning MSSA/MRSA screening (Methicillin-sensitive *S. aureus*); an intra-operative phase with several advices to observe during surgery, resumed in Box 2; and antibiotic therapy timing outlined in Box 3.

This protocol has been applied in a standardized way to all patients operated for breast cancer and reconstructed using prosthetic implants, from June 2020 on. We considered the type of mastectomy; the overall duration of the surgical procedure; eventual use of acellular dermal matrices; post-operative complications; the need for revision surgeries.

Box 1. Prevention Protocol for SSIs—Pre-operative phase.

PRE-OPERATIVE PHASE
Screening for MSSA/MRSA (up to 6 weeks prior to surgery): - Nostrils swab - Cutaneous (axillary and perineal) swab Decolonization: - Body washing with chlorhexidine 4% (daily, from 3 days before surgery) - Intraoral washing with chlorhexidine oral rinse (on the day of surgery) Eradication if tested positive for MSSA: - Body washing with chlorhexidine 4% (daily, from 3 days before surgery) - Mupirocin 2% nasal ointment (applied three times daily, from 3 days before surgery) Eradication if tested positive for MRSA: - Body washing with chlorhexidine 4% (daily, from 5 days before surgery) - Mupirocin 2% nasal ointment (applied three times daily, from 5 days before surgery) - Re-screening 48–72 h after eradication protocol *
MSSA, Methicillin-sensitive *S. aureus*; MRSA, Methicillin-resistant *S. aureus*; SSIs, surgical site infections. * It is mandatory to have 3 negative screenings before surgery, done at a time frame of 7 days or more after the eradication protocol, which could be administered maximum twice; if the patient keeps being tested positive for MRSA, administer adequate intravenous antibiotic prophylaxis before surgery and if possible, isolate the patient.

Box 2. Prevention Protocol for SSIs—Intra-operative phase.

INTRA-OPERATIVE PHASE
- Surgical hand preparation with antimicrobial soap and water or alcohol-based hand rub before donning sterile gloves - Preparation of the skin prior to draping using 2% chlorhexidine with 70% isopropyl alcohol - Perform careful atraumatic pocket dissection and careful haemostasis - Change surgical gloves every 60' to 90' and before handling implants - Perform pocket irrigation * - Minimize implant open time to reduce contamination Use a "minimal or no touch" technique where possible - Use closed suction drains to reduce hematoma or seroma formation in selected cases, "tunneling" them into a subcutaneous plane - Warming devices should be used to prevent hypothermia - It is recommended to reduce the operating time - Laminar airflow ventilation system
* There is a paucity of data supporting one form of washout to another. At our institution, we perform pocket and implant washing with antiseptic antibacterial 50% betadine double-antibiotic solution.

Box 3. Prevention Protocol for SSIs—Antibiotic prophylaxis.

ANTIBIOTIC PROPHYLAXIS
Intravenous antibiotic prophylaxis at the time of induction, for every patient:
- Cefazolin 2 g;
- OR Clindamycin 600 mg, if penicillin or cephalosporins allergies;
- Vancomycin 15 mg/kg + Gentamicin 3 mg/kg, if patient positive for MRSA
Intravenous 24-h multiple-dose antibiotic prophylaxis:
- Cefazolin 1 g q8hr;
- OR Clindamycin 600 mg q8hr, if penicillin or cephalosporins allergies;
Prolonged post-operative antibiotic prophylaxis, in high-risk patients:
- Cefalexin 500 P.O. q6hr;
- OR Clindamycin 300 mg P.O. q8hr, if penicillin or cephalosporins allergies
P.O., oral administration.

The collected data were inserted and analyzed in two different databases: the retrospective included patients who developed SSI between January 2007 and June 2020 and the prospective which included patients from June to September 2020.

The data were collected and managed using Microsoft Excel (Microsoft Office 365). Descriptive statistic was performed using IBM SPSS Version 24.

3. Results

3.1. Retrospective Analysis

In the period between January 2007 and June 2020, a total of 756 patients underwent surgical procedures involving prosthetic material for breast reconstruction. Twenty-six patients were diagnosed with SSI during the first year of follow-up after surgery.

Two out of 26 were Superficial incisional SSIs (7.7%); 24 out of 26 were Deep incisional SSIs (92.3%). No Organ or Space SSIs were reported (see Table 1).

Table 1. SSIs' characteristics.

Variable	No. (%)
SSI classification	
Superficial incisional SSI	2 (7.7)
Deep incisional SSI	24 (92.3)
Organ or space SSI	0 (0)
SSI onset	
Early	15 (57.7)
Late	11 (42.3)
Pathogens	
S. aureus	7 (26.9)
S. epidermidis	8 (30.8)
Coagulase-negative staphylococci	2 (7.7)
Gram-negative bacteria	5 (19.3)
Actinobacteria	2 (7.7)
Fungi	1 (3.8)
No bacterial growth	1 (3.8)
Outcome	
Need for revision surgery	14 (53.8)
Only antibiotic therapy	12 (46.2)

SSI, Surgical site infection.

Fifteen out of 26 SSIs had an early (within 30 days from surgery) onset (57.7%), 11 out of 26 SSIs had a late (between 31 days and 1 year after surgery) onset (42.3%); the median onset of SSI was 19 days after surgery.

Clinical signs, related to the onset of SSI, have not uniformly manifested in all 26 patients: we recorded local signs, such as redness, tenderness, warmth, or swelling in 24 out of 26 patients; fever was reported in 10 cases; purulent fluid discharge was reported in 7 cases. Clinical signs were supported by the evidence of inflammation markers increase C-reactive Protein (CPR) or Erythrocyte sedimentation rate (ESR) in 25 cases.

The organisms isolated from microbial cultures included: *S. aureus* was in 7 cases; *S. epidermidis* in 8 cases; other Coagulase-negative staphylococci in 2 cases; Gram-negative bacteria in 5 cases, Actinobacteria in two cases, and Fungi in one case. One patient had cultures done, but with negative bacterial growth.

At first, an empiric IV antibiotic treatment with βlactam ± inhibitor or Clindamycin was given in all SSIs pending cultures of wound's swab or periprosthetic fluid collection. Later, targeted antibiotic therapy was administered: in 12 cases (46.2%), this was sufficient to contain and resolve the infection; in the remaining 14 cases (53.8%), a revision surgery was performed.

3.2. Preliminary Analysis after the Introduction of the Prevention Protocol for SSIs

From June 2020 to September 2020, we prospectively enrolled 22 patients. Nine cases were bilateral. Altogether, we treated 31 breasts. In two of the bilateral cases, a contralateral breast surgery for symmetry was performed without using implant (one breast reduction and one mastopexy). We placed a total of 29 prosthetic devices (tissue expanders or implants). Twelve cases were immediate breast reconstructions after mastectomy, involving either tissue expander or implant; 10 cases were tissue expander (or implant) replacements with potential contralateral breast surgery to achieve symmetry. Mean mastectomy flap thickness in patients undergoing immediate breast reconstruction was 16.2 mm (range, 4.7 to 36.4). Three out of 12 patients had poor implant flap coverage (flap thickness < 10 mm); 6 out of 12 had medium-thickness flap coverage (flap thickness between 10 and 20 mm); 3 out of 12 patients had good implant flap coverage (flap thickness > 20 mm). Mean implant ($n = 20$) size was 390 cc (range, 140 to 690 cc); mean tissue expander ($n = 9$) volume was 428 cc (range, 250 to 650 cc), and mean intra-operative inflated volume was 40% (range, 18 to 72%). More surgical details are reported in Table 2.

Table 2. Surgical details.

Patient	Timing	Side	Left Side	Axilla	Reconstruction	Anatomical Plane	ADM	Right Side	Axilla	Reconstruction	Anatomical Plane	ADM	Operative Time (min)
1	IBR	Bilat	NSM	LNB	TE	Sub-pec	-	NSM	-	TE	Sub-pec	-	295
2	IBR	Bilat	NSM	-	Implant	Pre-pec	Braxon®	NSM	-	Implant	Pre-pec	Braxon®	226
3	IBR	Left	SSM	LFD	TE	Sub-pec	-	-	-	-	-	-	187
4	RPS	Bilat	-	-	TE to Impl	Sub-pec	-	-	-	TE to Impl	Sub-pec	-	189
5	IBR	Right	-	-	-	-	-	NSM	LNB	TE	Sub-pec	-	215
6	IBR	Left	SSM	LND	TE	Sub-pec	-	-	-	-	-	-	188
7	IBR	Left	SSM	LNB	TE	Sub-pec	-	-	-	-	-	-	174
8	IBR	Left	NSM	LNB	TE	Sub-pec	-	-	-	-	-	-	183
9	RPS	Left	-	-	TE to Impl	Pre-pec	-	-	-	-	-	-	70
10	RPS	Bilat	-	-	TE to Impl	Sub-pec	-	-	-	Breast Aug	Pre-pec	-	83
11	RPS	Right	-	-	-	-	-	-	-	TE to Impl	Sub-pec	-	130
12	RPS	Left	-	-	TE to Impl	Sub-pec	-	-	-	-	-	-	60
13	RPS	Left	-	-	TE to Impl	Pre-pec	-	-	-	-	-	-	70
14	IBR	Bilat	NSM	-	Implant	Pre-pec	Braxon®	NSM	LNB	Implant	Pre-pec	Braxon®	248
15	IBR	Right	-	-	-	-	-	SSM	LND	TE	Sub-pec	-	300
16	RPS	Bilat	-	-	Impl to Impl	Sub-pec	-	-	-	Mastopexy	-	-	150
17	IBR	Right	-	-	-	-	-	SSM	LND	Implant	Pre-pec	Braxon®	180
18	RPS	Bilat	-	-	Aug-Pexy	Pre-pec	-	-	-	TE to Impl	Sub-pec	-	170
19	IBR	Bilat	NSM	-	Implant	Pre-pec	Braxon®	NSM	LNB	Implant	Pre-pec	Braxon®	270
20	IBR	Right	-	-	-	-	-	SSM	LNB	TE	Sub-pec	-	190
21	RPS	Left	-	-	TE to Implant	Sub-pec	-	-	-	-	-	-	65
22	RPS	Bilat	-	-	TE to Implant	Sub-pec	-	-	-	Breast Red	-	-	162

IBR, Immediate Breast Reconstruction; RPS, Replacement surgery; NSM, Nipple-sparing mastectomy; SSM, Skin-sparing mastectomy; LNB, Lymph node biopsy; LND, Lymph node dissection; TE, Tissue expander; TE to Impl, Tissue expander replacement with Implant; Impl to Impl, Implant replacement with Implant; Breast Aug, Breast Augmentation; Aug-Pexy, Mastopexy with breast augmentation; Breast Red, Breast Reduction; Pre-pec, pre-pectoral plane; Sub-pec, sub-pectoral plane; ADM, Acellular dermal matrix.

Mean age at surgery was 54.9 years (range, 28 to 75 years). Most patients were nonsmokers (90.9%). A total of 5 patients (22.7%) had risk factors such as diabetes mellitus, obesity, or immunosuppression status; only 1 patient had previous breast radiation therapy or postmastectomy radiation therapy. BRCA1 or BRCA2 positivity was noted in 3 patients (13.6%) (Table 3).

Table 3. Patients' demographics.

Variable	No. (%)
Mean Age	54.9
Smoking	
Current smoker	2 (9.1)
Nonsmoker	20 (90.9)
Comorbidities	
Obesity (BMI $\geq$ 30 kg/m^2)	1 (4.5)
DM	3 (13.6)
IS	2 (9.1)
BRCA+	3 (13.6)
Previous XRT	1 (4.5)
MSSA carrier	3 (13.6)
MRSA carrier	0 (0)

BMI, Body Mass Index; DM, Diabetes Mellitus; BRCA, Breast-Related Cancer Antigens; XRT, Radiation therapy; IS, Immunosuppression status; MSSA, Methicillin-sensitive *S. aureus*; MRSA, Methicillin-resistant *S. aureus*.

Three out of 22 patients (13.6%) tested positive for MSSA (1 patient was nasal carrier, 1 patient was cutaneous carrier, 1 was both nasal and cutaneous carrier) and underwent eradication treatment. No patients in the study tested positive for MRSA.

The mean follow-up period was 85.4 days (range, 33 to 129). At the moment, none of the enrolled patients had early post-operative SSIs.

Table 4 reports infection rates (%) from 2007 to 2020: it shows how the (early) infection rates dropped to 0% after the introduction of the Prevention Protocol for SSIs in June 2020. The results of late SSI for the year 2020 at this moment are unavailable.

Table 4. Infection rates.

Year	SSI (n)	Patients (n)	SSI %
2007	0	21	0
2008	0	17	0
2009	2	18	11.11
2010	2	17	11.76
2011	1	33	3.03
2012	4	56	7.14
2013	3	56	5.36
2014	2	48	4.17
2015	3	67	4.48
2016	1	76	1.32
2017	3	94	3.19
2018	2	105	1.90
2019	2	101	1.98
January–May 2020	1	47	2.13
June–September 2020	**0**	**22**	**0**

Table 4. Surgical site infection (SSI) rates. Please note that the infection rate for the year 2020 considers only early surgical site infections. Highlighted in bold is the period from June to September 2020 related to the introduction of the Prevention Protocol for SSIs.

4. Discussion

Surgical site infection (SSI) is one of the most common healthcare-associated infections (HAIs). SSI is a significant surgical complication in prosthetic breast reconstruction as it may lead to a longer hospital stay with increasing costs for the national health system. For the patient, it is a devastating complication when it ends with the loss of reconstruction.

There is a lack of evidence-based benefits of SSI prevention strategies in implant-based breast reconstruction. Breast implant infection rates reported in the literature range from less than 1% up to 43% [1–4]. This variability can be explained in part by the lack of a standardized definition. Moreover, infection rates are not always well documented. All these make performing of sufficiently powered studies to provide meaningful results difficult.

Over the years, different techniques have been introduced in order to improve aesthetic and functional results in breast reconstruction. The use of prosthetic breast reconstruction has risen significantly, becoming the most frequent choice [20,21].

Patients undergoing implant-based breast reconstruction are subject to a range of infection prevention measures which are not standardized across institutions or countries. Actions to reduce SSIs have varying degrees of evidence for their efficacy, ranging from expert opinion to randomized trials, and are extremely debated.

Not unexpectedly, many hot topics and controversies in this field have emerged, including antibiotic prophylaxis, management of implant and pocket, early treatment of SSI.

Our study aimed to compare the infection rates related to implant-based breast reconstruction carried out at the Plastic and Reconstructive Surgery Unit of ASUGI—Trieste to those reported in the literature.

We reported a decreasing trend in SSIs' rate over time (range, 0% to 11.76%). Since the introduction of the Prevention Protocol for SSIs in June 2020, no case of early infection occurred among patients undergoing implant-based breast reconstruction was noticed. Late infections require a one-year follow-up, so the results of the prospective study cannot be compared to the retrospective ones.

However, we remain confident that the decreasing trend of infection rate could continue and stand as close as possible to zero.

Our study reports 2 Superficial incisional SSIs (7.7%), 24 Deep incisional SSIs (92.3%), and no Organ or Space SSI. This trend reflects what has been reported in most of the studies and points out how SSIs related to prosthetic breast reconstruction rarely involve any area of the body other than skin, muscle, and surrounding tissue involved in the surgery [12].

Most early SSIs and implant failures are associated with endogenous skin flora that colonize the nipple, including *S. aureus*, streptococci, and lactobacilli species [13]. Our findings support this data, as we frequently isolated staphylococci from microbial cultures; *S. aureus* was identified in 7 cases; *S. epidermidis* in 8 cases; and other Coagulase-negative staphylococci in 2 cases.

Although most SSIs are generally thought to occur within a month, some occur later, even after many years [22,23]. We reported 42.3% of SSIs with late onset, occurring between 31 days to 1 year after surgery. We agree with Sinha et al. who, in 2017, showed, in a prospective multi-center trial, that 47–71% of total SSI complications occur as late infections and criticized data collection limited to a 30 day period following surgery, which significantly underestimates the risk of actual SSI in implant-based reconstructions [24].

The clinical spectrum of breast implant infection is highly variable. In our series, clinical signs have not uniformly manifested in all 26 cases: we recorded local signs, such as redness, tenderness, warmth, or swelling in 24 out of 26 patients; fever was reported in 10 cases; and purulent fluid discharge in 7 cases. Clinical signs were supported by a raise of the inflammation markers (CRP or ESR) in 25 cases.

The management of breast implant infection often involves tissue expander or implant removal and targeted intravenous antibiotic therapy for up to two weeks for common infections. Positioning of a new implant following removal can be attempted within 3–6 months, although this may not be possible in cases involving chest wall radiotherapy. In order to attempt salvage of prosthetic reconstruction, systemic antibiotics without implant removal may be successful in a subset of patients with mild SSIs [25,26].

SSIs in our series were managed in the first instance with empiric βlactam ± inhibitor or Clindamycin IV antibiotics treatment pending cultures of wound's swab or periprosthetic fluid collection. Later, targeted antibiotic therapy was administered. Our data showed a 46.2% prosthesis salvage rate for SSIs that were treated with parenteral antibiotics only. Our salvage rate is comparable to those reported by other authors who have employed both surgical and medical treatments [27–29].

New antimicrobials, lipoglycopeptides, like dalbavancin, are long-acting antibiotics with potential for less frequent administration [30].

Patients undergoing implant-based breast reconstruction are exposed to a range of pre-operative, intra-operative, and post-operative prevention measures which are not standardized across institutions or countries, and which have varying degrees of evidence for their efficacy, ranging from expert opinion to randomized trials.

We created a standardized protocol for prevention of SSIs, based on international guidelines and evidence reported in the literature. We believe that it could be the starting point for further studies in the field of breast reconstruction. Only by creating a common pathway with standardized pre, intra and postoperative steps, we can study large populations, allowing more robust statistical analysis of complications and outcomes in breast reconstruction surgery.

Regarding the pre-operative management, MSSA and MRSA screening with appropriate treatment of carriers before surgery is recommended by several studies. General population carriage rates for *S. Aureus* are as high as 37.2%, and a carrier has a 7.1 relative risk of subsequently developing a related infection [14]. Our preliminary data show 13.6% MSSA carriage rate. Each patient underwent eradication treatment before surgery. No patients in the study tested positive for MRSA. Clearly, considering the commitment that requires a screening path, both in terms of personnel and materials, periodic revaluations will be necessary for a cost-benefit analysis, also based on the local prevalence of *S. Aureus*.

The retrospective nature of the analysis that was performed on infection rates at our institution has not allowed us to thoroughly analyze the risk factors involved. However, the data collection form that we have introduced along with the prevention protocol for SSIs will allow us to prospectively study the potential risk factors for each complication related to implant-based reconstruction.

Among these complications, SSI can cause devastating reconstructive failures in implant-based breast reconstructions; for this reason, the need for antibiotic prophylaxis remains one of the most debated topics. There is no consensus regarding the right duration of antibiotic prophylaxis after implant-based reconstruction, and whether it should be continued after surgery in the presence of a drain into the implant pocket or in selected high-risk patients (e.g., patients who had diabetes or recent radiation therapy).

Developing our protocol, we reviewed international guidelines [31,32], systematic reviews, and studies with high levels of evidence [17,33–41]. Prior to June 2020, all patients were subjected to prolonged antibiotic administration until drains removal. From June 2020, to all patients undergoing implant-based breast reconstruction we administered antibiotic prophylaxis extended to 24 h or longer in those patients deemed "high risk" for SSI, and as already pointed out, no case of infection occurred among them.

In clinical practice, there is a lack of standardization in terms of pre-, intra-, and post-operative care for patients undergoing implant-based breast reconstruction. Our new protocol shows excellent preliminary results in term of infection prevention.

Despite the limited sample size and relatively short prospective follow-up period not allowing for a statistically significant analysis of its effectiveness, the preliminary data, showing absence of early SSIs, could potentially lead to a decreasing trend also of late infection rates.

5. Conclusions

SSI is clearly a significant surgical complication in implant-based breast reconstruction as it may lead to a longer hospital stay with increasing costs for the national health system, and it may result in the loss of reconstruction, a potentially devastating complication for the patient.

Infection rates at our institution are comparable to those reported in the literature and show a decreasing trend over time. Additionally, since the introduction of the Prevention Protocol for SSIs in June 2020, no cases of infection were reported among patients undergoing implant-based breast reconstruction. As mentioned above, despite the limited sample size and relatively short prospective follow-up period not allowing for a statistically significant analysis of the effectiveness of this protocol, the preliminary data, with absence of early SSIs, could show a promising decreasing trend also of late SSI infection rates. We further believe that creation of a common shared pathway, with standardized pre-, intra-, and post-operative steps, represents the cornerstone for a valid and efficient treatment for the patient; moreover, it is also the starting point to carry out more robust analysis of complications and outcomes in implant-based breast reconstruction.

Author Contributions: Conceptualization, G.P. (Giuseppe Pizzolato), A.F. and Z.M.A.; methodology, G.P. (Giovanni Papa); software, G.P. (Giovanni Papa); validation, G.P. (Giovanni Papa), A.F. and Z.M.A.; formal analysis, G.P. (Giuseppe Pizzolato); investigation, G.P. (Giuseppe Pizzolato) and N.R.; resources, G.P. (Giovanni Papa); data curation, G.P. (Giuseppe Pizzolato) and A.F.; writing—original draft preparation, G.P. (Giuseppe Pizzolato) and A.F.; writing—review and editing, A.F., C.S. and Z.M.A.; visualization, V.R.; supervision, G.P. (Giovanni Papa) and Z.M.A.; project administration, G.P. (Giovanni Papa). All authors have read and agreed to the published version of the manuscript.

Institutional Review Board Statement: The study was conducted according to the guidelines of the Declaration of Helsinki.

Informed Consent Statement: Informed consent was obtained from all subjects involved in the study.

Conflicts of Interest: The authors declare no conflict of interest.

References

1. Ooi, A.S.H.; Song, D.H. Reducing infection risk in implant-based breast reconstruction surgery: Challenges and solutions. *Breast Cancer Targets Ther.* **2016**, *8*, 161–172.
2. Alderman, A.K.; Wilkins, E.G.; Kim, H.M.; Lowery, J.C. Complications in postmastectomy breast reconstruction: Two-year results of the Michigan breast reconstruction outcome study. *Plast. Reconstr. Surg.* **2002**, *109*, 2265–2274. [CrossRef] [PubMed]
3. Peled, A.W.; Itakura, K.; Foster, R.D.; Hamolsky, D.; Tanaka, J.; Ewing, C.; Alvarado, M.; Esserman, L.J.; Hwang, E.S. Impact of chemotherapy on postoperative complications after mastectomy and immediate breast reconstruction. *Arch Surg.* **2010**, *145*, 880–885. [CrossRef]
4. Azouz, V.; Mirhaidari, S.; Wagner, D.S. Defining Infection in Breast Reconstruction. *Ann. Plast. Surg.* **2018**, *80*, 587–591. [CrossRef] [PubMed]
5. Horan, T.C.; Gaynes, R.P.; Martone, W.J.; Jarvis, W.R.; Emori, T.G. CDC Definitions of Nosocomial Surgical Site Infections, 1992: A Modification of CDC Definitions of Surgical Wound Infections. *Infect. Control Hosp. Epidemiol.* **1992**, *13*, 606–608. [CrossRef] [PubMed]
6. Colwell, A.S.; Tessler, O.; Lin, A.M.; Liao, E.; Winograd, J.; Cetrulo, C.L.; Tang, R.; Smith, B.L.; Austen, W.G., Jr. Breast reconstruction following nipplesparing mastectomy: Predictors of complications, reconstruction outcomes, and 5-year trends. *Plast. Reconstr. Surg.* **2014**, *133*, 496–506. [CrossRef]
7. Antony, A.K.; McCarthy, C.M.; Cordeiro, P.G.; Mehrara, B.J.; Pusic, A.L.; Teo, E.H.; Arriaga, A.F.; Disa, J.J. Acellular human dermis implantation in 153 immediate two-stage TE breast reconstructions: Determining the incidence and significant predictors ofcomplications. *Plast. Reconstr. Surg.* **2010**, *125*, 1606–1614. [CrossRef]
8. Voineskos, S.H.; Frank, S.G.; Cordeiro, P.G. Breast reconstruction following conservative mastectomies: Predictors of complications and outcomes. *Gland Surg.* **2015**, *4*, 484–496. [PubMed]
9. Nahabedian, M.Y.; Tsangaris, T.; Momen, B.; Manson, P.N. Infectious complications following breast reconstruction with expanders and implants. *Plast. Reconstr. Surg.* **2003**, *112*, 467–476. [CrossRef] [PubMed]
10. Liu, A.S.; Kao, H.K.; Reish, R.G.; Hergrueter, C.A.; May, J.W.; Guo, L. Postoperative Complications in Prosthesis-Based Breast Reconstruction Using Acellular Dermal Matrix. *Plast. Reconstr. Surg.* **2011**, *127*, 1755–1762. [CrossRef]
11. Francis, S.H.; Ruberg, R.L.; Stevenson, K.B.; Beck, C.E.; Ruppert, A.S.; Harper, J.T.; Boehmler, J.H., IV; Miller, M.J. Independent risk factors for infection in tissue expander breast reconstruction. *Plast. Reconstr. Surg.* **2009**, *124*, 1790–1796. [CrossRef]
12. Culver, D.H.; Horan, T.C.; Gaynes, R.P.; Martone, W.J.; Jarvis, W.R.; Emori, T.G.; Banerjee, S.N.; Edwards, J.R.; Tolson, J.S.; Henderson, T.S.; et al. Surgical wound infection rates by wound class, operative procedure, and patient risk index. *Am. J. Med.* **1991**, *91*, S152–S157.

13. Throckmorton, A.D.; Baddour, L.M.; Hoskin, T.L.; Boughey, J.C.; Degnim, A.C. Microbiology of surgical site infections complicating breast surgery. *Surg. Infect.* **2010**, *11*, 355–359. [CrossRef] [PubMed]
14. Kluytmans, J.; van Belkum, A.; Verbrugh, H. Nasal carriage of Staphylococcus aureus: Epidemiology, underlying mechanisms, and associated risks. *Clin. Microbiol. Rev.* **1997**, *10*, 505–520. [CrossRef]
15. National Nosocomial Infections Surveillance System. National Nosocomial Infections Surveillance (NNIS) System Report, data summary from January 1992 through June 2004, issued October 2004. *Am. J. Infect. Control.* **2004**, *32*, 470–485. [CrossRef]
16. WHO. Summary of a systematic review on decolonization with mupirocin ointment with or without chlorhexidine gluconate body wash for the prevention of S. aureus infection in nasal carriers undergoing surgery. In *Surgical Site Infection Prevention Guidelines*; WHO: Geneva, Switzerland, 2018.
17. Pan, A.; Cappelli, V.; Parenti, M.; Pantosti, A.; Pompa, M.G.; Salcuni, P.; Moro, M.L. *Ministero della Salute. Raccomandazioni sul Controllo della Diffusione Nosocomiale dello Staphylococcus Aureus Resistente alla Meticillina (MRSA)*; Maggio: Bologna, Italy, 2011. Available online: http://www.salute.gov.it/imgs/C_17_pagineAree_648_listaFile_itemName_0_file.pdf (accessed on 30 December 2020).
18. Dancey, A.; Nassimizadeh, A.; Levick, P. Capsular contracture e what are the risk factors? A 14-year series of 1400 consecutive augmentations. *J. Plast. Reconstr. Aesthet. Surg.* **2012**, *65*, 213–218. [CrossRef] [PubMed]
19. Barr, S.P.; Topps, A.R.; Barnes, N.L.; Henderson, J.; Hignett, S.; Teasdale, R.L.; McKenna, A.; Harvey, J.R.; Kirwan, C.C. A Review of the Surgical Evidence, Guidelines and a Checklist. *Eur. J. Surg. Oncol.* **2016**, *42*, 591–603. [CrossRef]
20. Ribuffo, D.; Berna, G.; De Vita, R.; Di Benedetto, G.; Cigna, E.; Greco, M.; Valdatta, L.; Onesti, M.G.; Lo Torto, F.; Marcasciano, M.; et al. Dual-Plane Retro-pectoral Versus Pre-pectoral DTI Breast Reconstruction: An Italian Multicenter Experience. *Aesthetic Plast Surg.* **2020**. [CrossRef] [PubMed]
21. Sisti, A.; Huayllani, M.T.; Boczar, D.; Restrepo, D.J.; Spaulding, A.C.; Emmanuel, G.; Bagaria, S.P.; McLaughlin, S.A.; Parker, A.S.; Forte, A.J. Breast cancer in women: A descriptive analysis of the national cancer database. *Acta Biomed.* **2020**, *91*, 332–341. [PubMed]
22. Bennett, K.G.; Qi, J.; Kim, H.M.; Hamill, J.B.; Pusic, A.L.; Wilkins, E.G. Comparison of 2-Year Complication Rates Among Common Techniques for Postmastectomy Breast Reconstruction. *JAMA Surg.* **2018**, *153*, 901–908. [CrossRef]
23. Washer, L.L.; Gutowski, K. Breast implant infections. *Infect. Dis. Clin. N. Am.* **2012**, *26*, 111–125. [CrossRef] [PubMed]
24. Sinha, I.; Pusic, A.L.; Wilkins, E.G.; Hamill, J.B.; Chen, X.; Kim, H.M.; Guldbrandsen, G.; Chun, Y.S. Late Surgical-Site Infection in Immediate Implant-Based Breast Reconstruction. *Plast. Reconstr. Surg.* **2017**, *139*, 20–28. [CrossRef]
25. Spear, S.L.; Howard, M.A.; Boehmler, J.H.; Ducic, I.; Low, M.; Abbruzzesse, M.R. The infected or exposed breast implant: Management and treatment strategies. *Plast. Reconstr. Surg.* **2004**, *113*, 1634–1644. [CrossRef]
26. Halvorson, E.G.; Disa, J.J.; Mehrara, B.J.; Burkey, B.A.; Pusic, A.L.; Cordeiro, P.G. Outcome following remocal of infected tissue expanders in breast reconstruction: A 10-year experience. *Ann. Plast. Surg.* **2007**, *59*, 131–136. [CrossRef]
27. Reish, R.G.; Damjanovic, B.; Austen, W.G., Jr.; Winograd, J.; Liao, E.C.; Cetrulo, C.L.; Balkin, D.M.; Colwell, A.S. Infection following implant-based reconstruction in 1952 consecutive breast reconstructions: Salvage rates and predictors of success. *Plast. Reconstr. Surg.* **2013**, *131*, 1223–1230. [CrossRef]
28. Song, J.H.; Kim, Y.S.; Jung, B.K.; Lee, D.W.; Song, S.Y.; Roh, T.S.; Lew, D.H. Salvage of infected breast implants. *Arch. Plast. Surg.* **2017**, *44*, 516–522. [CrossRef]
29. Ozturk, C.; Ozturk, C.N.; Platek, M.; Soucise, A.; Laub, P.; Morin, N.; Lohman, R.; Moon, W. Management of Expander- and Implant-Associated Infections in Breast Reconstruction. *Aesthet. Plast. Surg.* **2020**, *44*, 2075–2082. [CrossRef]
30. Bassetti, M.; Peghin, M.; Carnelutti, A.; Righi, E. The role of dalbavancin in skin and soft tissue infections. *Curr. Opin. Infect. Dis.* **2018**, *31*, 141–147. [CrossRef] [PubMed]
31. *Global Guidelines for the Prevention of Surgical Site Infection*; WHO: Geneva, Switzerland, 2018; Available online: https://www.who.int/gpsc/ssi-prevention-guidelines/en/ (accessed on 30 December 2020).
32. Breast reconstruction with expanders and Implants. In *Evidence-Based Clinical Practice Guideline*; American Society of Plastic Surgeons: Arlington Heights, IL, USA, 2013.
33. Potter, S.; Conroy, E.J.; Cutress, R.I.; Williamson, P.R.; Whisker, L.; Thrush, S.; Skillman, J.; Barnes, N.L.; Mylvaganam, S.; Teasdale, E.; et al. Short-term safety outcomes of mastectomy and immediate implant-based breast reconstruction with and without mesh (iBRA): A multicentre, prospective cohort study. *Lancet Oncol.* **2019**, *20*, 254–266. [CrossRef]
34. Mylvaganam, S.; Conroy, E.J.; Williamson, P.R.; Barnes, N.L.; Cutress, R.I.; Gardiner, M.D.; Jain, A.; Skillman, J.M.; Thrush, S.; Whisker, L.J.; et al. Adherence to best practice consensus guidelines for implant-based breast reconstruction: Results from the iBRA national practice questionnaire survey. *Eur. J. Surg. Oncol.* **2018**, *44*, 708–716. [CrossRef] [PubMed]
35. Dave, R.; O'Connell, R.; Rattay, T.; Tolkien, Z.; Barnes, N.; Skillman, J.; Williamson, P.; Conroy, E.; Gardiner, M.; Harnett, A.; et al. The iBRA-2 study: Protocol for a prospective national multicentre cohort study to evaluate the impact of immediate breast reconstruction on the delivery of adjuvant therapy. *BMJ Open* **2016**, *6*, e012678. [CrossRef]
36. O'Connell, R.L.; Rattay, T.; Dave, R.V.; Trickey, A.; Skillman, J.; Barnes, N.L.; Gardiner, M.; Harnett, A.; Potter, S.; Holcombe, C. The impact of immediate breast reconstruction on the time to delivery of adjuvant therapy: The iBRA-2 study. *Br. J. Cancer* **2019**, *120*, 883–895. [CrossRef]

37. Clayton, J.L.; Bazakas, A.; Lee, C.N.; Hultman, C.S.; Halvorson, E.G. Once is not enough: Withholding postoperative prophylactic antibiotics in prosthetic breast reconstruction is associated with an increased risk of infection. *Plast. Reconstr. Surg.* **2012**, *130*, 495–502. [CrossRef]
38. McCullough, M.C.; Chu, C.K.; Duggal, C.S.; Losken, A.; Carlson, G.W. Antibiotic prophylaxis and resistance in surgical site infection after immediate tissue expander reconstruction of the breast. *Ann. Plast. Surg.* **2016**, *77*, 501–505. [CrossRef] [PubMed]
39. Phillips, B.T.; Bishawi, M.; Dagum, A.B.; Khan, S.U.; Bui, D.T. A systematic review of antibiotic use and infection in breast reconstruction: What is the evidence? *Plast. Reconstr. Surg.* **2013**, *131*, 1–13. [CrossRef] [PubMed]
40. Phillips, B.T.; Bishawi, M.; Dagum, A.B.; Bui, D.T.; Khan, S.U. A systematic review of infection rates and associated antibiotic duration in acellular dermal matrix breast reconstruction. *Eplasty* **2014**, *14*, e42. [PubMed]
41. Phillips, B.T.; Fourman, M.S.; Bishawi, M.; Zegers, M.; O'Hea, B.J.; Ganz, J.C.; Huston, T.L.; Dagum, A.B.; Khan, S.U.; Bui, D.T. Are prophylactic postoperative antibiotics necessary for immediate breast reconstruction? Results of a prospective randomized clinical trial. *J. Am. Coll. Surg.* **2016**, *222*, 1116–1124. [CrossRef] [PubMed]

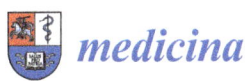

Article

Prediction of the Ideal Implant Size Using 3-Dimensional Healthy Breast Volume in Unilateral Direct-to-Implant Breast Reconstruction

Jeong-Hoon Kim, Jin-Woo Park and Kyong-Je Woo *

Department of Plastic and Reconstructive Surgery, Ewha Womans University Mokdong Hospital, College of Medicine, Ewha Womans University, 1071 Anyangcheon-ro, Yangcheon-gu, Seoul 07985, Korea; kimsbrothers@hanmail.net (J.-H.K.); burnscar@naver.com (J.-W.P.)
* Correspondence: economywoo@gmail.com

Received: 21 August 2020; Accepted: 18 September 2020; Published: 24 September 2020

Abstract: *Background and objectives:* There is no consensus regarding accurate methods for assessing the size of the implant required for achieving symmetry in direct-to-implant (DTI) breast reconstruction. The purpose of this study was to determine whether the ideal implant size could be estimated using 3D breast volume or mastectomy specimen weight, and to compare prediction performances between the two variables. *Materials and Methods*: Patients who underwent immediate DTI breast reconstruction from August 2017 to April 2020 were included in this study. Breast volumes were measured using 3D surface imaging preoperatively and at postoperative three months. Ideal implant size was calculated by correcting the used implant volume by the observed postoperative asymmetry in 3D surface imaging. Prediction models using mastectomy weight or 3D volume were made to predict the ideal implant volume. The prediction performance was compared between the models. *Results*: A total of 56 patients were included in the analysis. In correlation analysis, the volume of the implant used was significantly correlated with the mastectomy specimen weight ($R^2 = 0.810$) and the healthy breast volume ($R^2 = 0.880$). The mean ideal implant volume was 278 ± 123 cc. The prediction model was developed using the healthy breast volume: Implant volume (cc) = healthy breast volume × 0.78 + 26 cc ($R^2 = 0.900$). The prediction model for the ideal implant size using the 3D volume showed better prediction performance than that of using the mastectomy specimen weight ($R^2 = 0.900$ vs 0.759, $p < 0.001$). *Conclusions*: The 3D volume of the healthy breast is a more reliable predictor than mastectomy specimen weight to estimate the ideal implant size. The estimation formula obtained in this study may assist in the selection of the ideal implant size in unilateral DTI breast reconstruction.

Keywords: 3D breast volume; direct-to-implant breast reconstruction; estimation of ideal implant size

1. Introduction

Nipple sparing mastectomy (NSM) and direct-to-implant (DTI) breast reconstruction have been gaining popularity because it is oncologically safe, requires less surgery and fewer visits, and is more cost-effective than two-stage expander/implant reconstruction [1–3]. Surgeons choose the implants considering the weight of the resected breast tissue, the patient anatomy as assessed by subjective linear measurements, the surgeon's experience, and the availability of implants. However, linear measurements including the height, width, and projection of the breasts are insufficient to describe the breast shape and size accurately, and small measurement discrepancies may lead to variations in volumetric implant size estimation and potentially unacceptable asymmetry. Although various methods have been developed, there is no universally accepted standard method for determining breast volume and for choosing the optimal implant size for breast reconstruction.

In the last decade, advances in 3-dimensional surface imaging have produced techniques for handling vast data formats efficiently and generating precise 3-dimensional surface images [4–6]. The breast volume can be measured preoperatively using 3D surface imaging, and the 3D volumes are known to be significantly correlated with the mastectomy specimen weight [7]. Similar to the mastectomy specimen weight, the preoperative 3D volume of the breasts can assist the surgeon in calculating the ideal volume of the implant. However, there have been no guidelines developed regarding how to estimate ideal implant volume using 3D volume data of the breast. The purpose of this study was to determine whether the ideal implant size could be estimated using 3-dimensional breast volume or mastectomy specimen weight, and to compare prediction performances between these two variables.

2. Materials and Methods

2.1. Study Population and Data Collection

The study was conducted in accordance with the Declaration of Helsinki, and the protocol was approved by the institutional review board of Ewha Womans University Mokdong Hospital (No. 2020-07-046). Prospectively recorded data from consecutive patients who underwent immediate unilateral DTI reconstruction at a single institution between August 2017 and April 2020 were retrospectively reviewed. Patients who underwent bilateral breast reconstruction, simultaneous contralateral augmentation/reduction surgery, previous surgery on the affected breast side, and patients with incomplete records were excluded. Data on patient demographics, surgical procedures, mastectomy specimen weight, and implant size used were collected. Breast volumes were measured using 3D surface imaging preoperatively and at postoperative three months. The primary outcome was the ideal implant size, which was calculated by correcting the used implant volume by the observed postoperative asymmetry in 3D surface imaging. The independent variables were either the mastectomy specimen weight or the preoperative 3D volume of the healthy breast.

2.2. Method for 3-Dimensional Surface Imaging and Volume Extraction

Volumetric assessment of the breast was obtained using a Crisalix 3D® imaging scan (Crisalix, Lausanne, Switzerland). The Crisalix system is a cloud-based, 3-dimensional simulation program. 3D surface scanning was performed using a 3D sensor attached to a portable tablet to scan the patient's front and both sides in a standing position. The total time for each individual scan was a few seconds, and the total procedure time, including marking of breast landmarks, takes less than 10 s. All 3D scans were performed with the patient in the same position. Patients were scanned in a standing position with the back of the feet and the shoulders touching the wall, and arms abducted with both wrists placed on the hips of the patients.

Data from the 3-dimensional scan are uploaded and merged to generate a 3-dimensional surface image, which is then rendered. This software program can then generate the curvature of the simulated chest wall and the indicated breast boundary from the torso curved to match the real body shape and thereby calculate the volume of the 3D breast image [8]. After completing the 3-dimensional surface image, the volume of the breast soft tissue was measured with consideration of 3 mm skin thickness (Figure 1). Postoperatively, the 3D surface imaging was repeated to compare the volumes of the reconstructed and healthy breasts at three months postoperative follow-up using the same protocol.

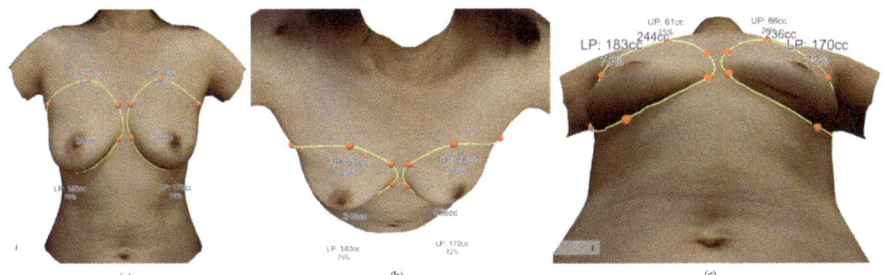

Figure 1. A case example of preoperative 3-D volumes of the breasts. (**a**) Anterior view. (**b**) Cephalic to caudal view. (**c**) Caudal to cephalic view.

2.3. Reconstruction after Nipple-Sparing Mastectomy

Oncologic surgeons performed the mastectomy, and the senior author (K.J.W.) performed all reconstructions. The implant size and type were determined by the surgeon considering the patient's breast dimensions, contralateral breast volume measured before surgery, and the resected mastectomy specimen weight to achieve symmetric breasts. The size of the implant used was determined after two or three temporary sizers were inserted and checking the breast symmetry by visual inspection and palpation. The implants were placed in the subpectoral or prepectoral spaces. In subpectoral DTI, an acellular dermal matrix (human cadaveric) of 6–8 × 16–18 cm size was used for inferior and lateral support and implant coverage. In prepectoral DTI, a 16 × 16 cm or 18 × 18 cm acellular dermal matrix was used to cover the implant.

2.4. Calculation of Ideal Implant Size

Because the implants used were not always the ideal size for symmetry in unilateral DTI breast reconstructions, an ideal implant size was calculated by correcting the used implant volume by the observed postoperative asymmetry in 3D surface imaging. The ideal implant volume = Inserted implant volume − β × (Surgical side breast volume − Contralateral side breast volume measured postoperatively at three months after surgery). The β was the slope of the linear regression model that was obtained using the preoperative breast volume as an independent variable and the inserted implant volume as the dependent variable. If the β was 0.7, a 100 cc increase of the breast volume resulted in a 70 cc increase of the implant volume in the linear regression model.

2.5. Statistical Analysis

The mean with standard deviation or median with interquartile range were used to summarize continuous variables based on the distribution of the data. Pearson correlation coefficients between implant size and morphological factors, including mastectomy specimen weight and healthy breast volume, were first examined to determine the most suitable references for implant size choice. Linear regression analysis was performed to develop formulas predicting the optimal inserted implant volume.

After calculation of the ideal implant sizes, linear regression models were used to develop formulas to predict the ideal implant volume for symmetry using mastectomy specimen weight and preoperative healthy breast volume as predictor variables. The prediction performances using the two predictor variables were compared. Residual analysis was performed to assess the appropriateness of the linear regression model. The statistical significance was determined by $p < 0.05$. All analyses were performed using SPSS version 23.0 (SPSS Inc., Chicago, IL, USA).

3. Results

3.1. Patient Demographics and Operative Data

A total of 56 patients undergoing immediate unilateral DTI reconstruction were included in the analysis. The patients' mean age was 47.95 ± 8.44 years (IQR, 43.5–52.3) with a mean BMI of 22.77 ± 2.50 kg/m^2 (IQR, 20.92–24.25). Nipple-sparing mastectomy was performed in 85.7% (48 of 56 patients), and skin-sparing mastectomy was performed in the remaining cases. Prepectoral placement of the implant was performed in 46.4%, and subpectoral placement was performed in 53.6%. The mean preoperative volume of the affected breast was 318 ± 154 cc (IQR, 194–408) and that of the contralateral unaffected breast was 323 ± 150 cc (IQR, 203–380). The mean mastectomy specimen weight was 287 ± 128 g (IQR, 181–348) and the mean volume of inserted implant was 288 ± 107 cc (IQR, 200–375) (Table 1).

Table 1. Clinical and surgical characteristics.

No. of patients	56
Age, mean ± SD, yr	47.95 ± 8.44
BMI, mean ± SD, kg/m^2	22.77 ± 2.50
Cancer laterality	
No. of right (%)	35 (62.5)
No. of left (%)	21 (37.5)
Mastectomy type	
No. of nipple-sparing (%)	48 (85.7)
No. of skin-sparing (%)	8 (14.3)
Mastectomy specimen weight, mean ± SD, g	287.6 ± 128.2
Inserted implant volume, mean ± SD, cc	287.5 ± 107.0
Inserted ADM size, mean ± SD, cm^2	204.0 ± 82.9
Preoperative volume of the breasts	
Pre-operative volume of affected breast, mean ± SD, cc	317.6 ± 154.3
Pre-operative volume of contralateral unaffected breast, mean ± SD, cc	322.9 ± 150.0
Postoperative volume of the breasts	
Post-operative volume of affected breast, mean ± SD, cc	336.8 ± 147.8
Post-operative volume of contralateral unaffected breast, mean ± SD, cc	321.2 ± 161.1

SD, standard deviation; BMI, body mass index; ADM, acellular dermal matrix.

In the analysis of preoperative 3D volume of the healthy and affected breasts, mean volume differences of the breasts were 49.5 ± 39.8 cc (IQR, 23.0–76.0 cc) (Figure 2). The mean percentage of volume differences was 15.8 ± 13.4% (IQR, 8.5–23.1%), and 32.1% of the patients (18 of 56) had over 20% volume differences between the healthy and affected breasts.

3.2. Prediction Model for the Inserted Implant Volume

The Pearson correlation coefficient of the mastectomy specimen weight was 0.900 ($p < 0.001$). In the linear regression analysis, a prediction model was developed (Figure 3).

1. Inserted implant volume = 0.75 × mastectomy specimen weight (g) + 72 cc (R2 = 81.0%, $p < 0.001$).

The Pearson correlation coefficient of the healthy breast volume was 0.938 ($p < 0.001$). In the linear regression analysis, the inserted implant volume was better estimated with the model using healthy breast volume.

2. Inserted implant volume = 0.66 × healthy breast volume + 71 cc (R2 = 88.0%, $p < 0.001$).

The results of the residual analysis satisfied the assumptions of the linear regression models.

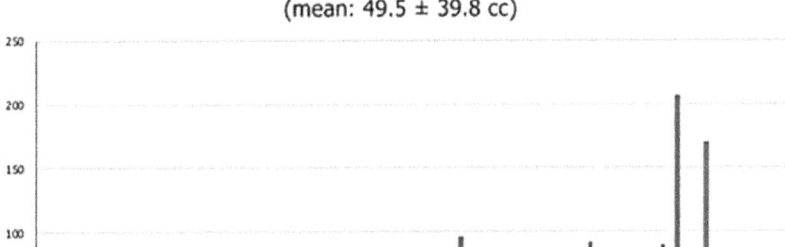

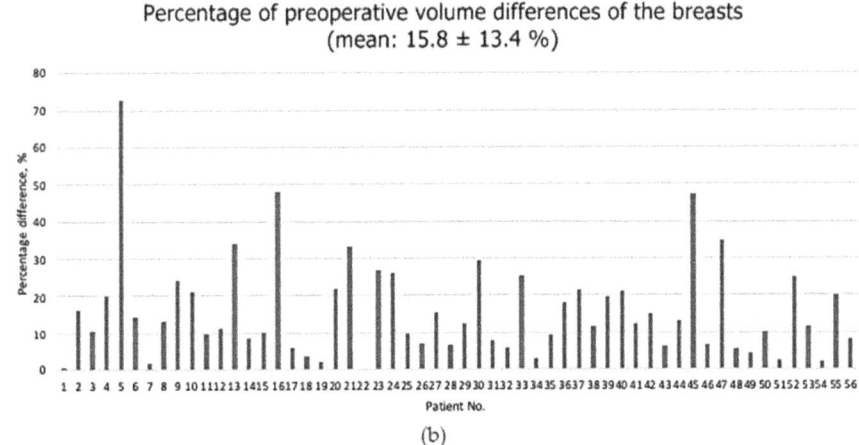

Figure 2. (a) Preoperative volume differences of the breasts. (b) Percentage of preoperative volume differences of the breasts. The percentage of volume differences were calculated by (1-reconstruction side breast volume/healthy breast volume) × 100.

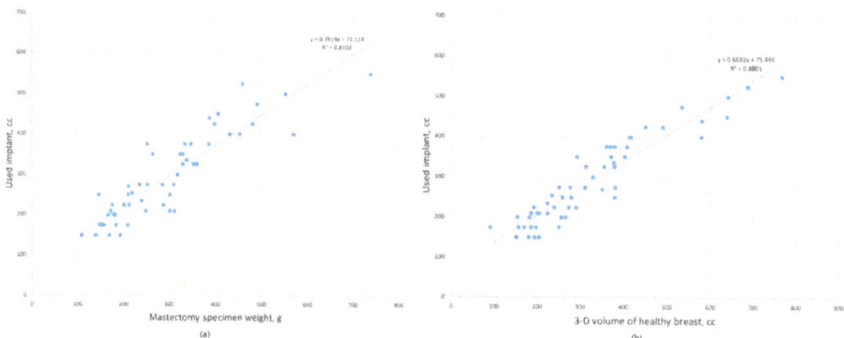

Figure 3. Predication model for inserted implant. (**a**) Scatterplot and the linear regression model using mastectomy specimen weight as a predictor variable. (**b**) Scatterplot and the linear regression model using 3-D volume of healthy breast as a predictor variable.

3.3. Prediction Model for Ideal Implant Volume

Because the inserted implant volume could not be considered as an ideal implant volume for symmetry, ideal implant volume was calculated by comparing the postoperative volumes of both breasts. The mean volume of the ideal implant size was 278 ± 123 cc (IQR, 181–338 cc). The prediction model of an ideal implant volume was as follows (Figure 4).

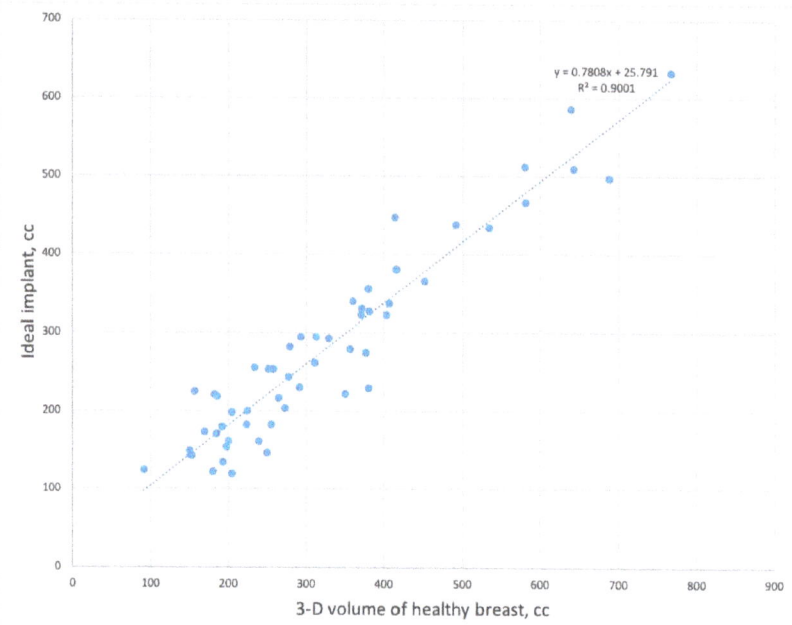

Figure 4. Predication model for ideal implant. Scatterplot and the linear regression model using 3-D volume of healthy breast as a predictor variable.

1. Mastectomy specimen weight as a predictor variable.

    Ideal implant volume = mastectomy specimen weight × 0.84 + 37 cc (R2 = 75.9%, $p < 0.001$).

2. Healthy breast volume as a predictor variable.

Ideal implant volume = healthy breast volume × 0.78 + 25 cc (R^2 = 90.0%, $p < 0.001$).

The results of the linear regression models showed that an ideal implant volume could be predicted by both healthy breast volume and mastectomy specimen weight. In terms of prediction performance, the ideal implant volume could be better estimated using the 3D volume of the healthy breast compared to the mastectomy specimen weight (coefficient of determination = 90.0% vs. 75.9%). The results of the residual analysis satisfied the assumptions of linear regression models.

4. Discussion

The selection of an ideal size of implant is crucial for achieving symmetry in immediate DTI breast reconstruction. The current study demonstrated that the ideal implant size could be estimated by a linear regression model using either mastectomy specimen weight ($p < 0.001$) or the 3D volume of the healthy breast ($p < 0.001$). Moreover, we found that the 3D volume could predict the ideal implant size more accurately than the mastectomy specimen weight (R^2 = 0.900 vs. 0.759).

Many surgeons subjectively evaluate the breast volumes and symmetry. However, subjective measurement of breast volume cannot be reliable and is not accurate [9]. Mastectomy specimen weight has been proposed to be used as a reference for the selection of ideal implant size [10–13]. The density of mastectomy specimen weight is known to be 1.06 g/mL [14]. However, the density of the breast is different among patients because the proportions of fibro-glandular tissue and fat tissue volume of the breast are different. The tumor itself can also change the density and weight of the affected breast.

Furthermore, innate breast asymmetry cannot be taken into account when using the mastectomy specimen as a reference to estimate the ideal implant size. Recently, Liu et al. found that the incidence of significant asymmetry of the breast mound was 94 percent [15]. We also found that most patients had innate asymmetry of their breast volumes. The mean percentage of volume differences was 15.8 ± 13.4% (IQR, 8.5–23.1%), and about one-third of the patients (18 of 56) had over 20% volume differences between the healthy and affected breasts in our study. Georgiou et al. reported that the implant size could be predicted by the mastectomy specimen weight using a linear regression model, but there were limitations since the coefficient of determination (R^2) was less that 0.5 (R = 0.66) [11].

2-dimensional images of CT or MRI and subsequent 3D reconstruction can be used for breast volume measurement [12,16–20]. However, 3D reconstruction of the 2D images are complex and need additional software. Moreover, it is not completely objective because boundary annotation of the breast tissue has to be performed manually or threshold of breast tissue has to be arbitrarily determined on the 2D images.

Recently, 3D surface imaging has gained acceptance in clinical use in breast surgery [4–6]. 3D surface imaging has been used for the selection of implant size and for creating simulations for augmentation mammoplasty [21–24]. Yip et al. reported that breast volume could be measured by 3D surface imaging (Pearson's correlation, R = 0.95, $p < 0.001$) [7]. Roostaeian et al. evaluated the accuracy of the 3D surface imaging and reported that preoperative simulation by 3D surface imaging can predict postoperative breast volume with more than 90% accuracy [25]. Previous studies have suggested the potential use of 3D surface imaging for measuring the breast volume for selection of the ideal implant size in DTI breast reconstructions. We found that the 3D volume of the healthy breast measured by 3D surface imaging could be used for estimation of the ideal implant size. We also demonstrated that the 3D volume of the healthy breast showed better prediction performance than the mastectomy specimen weight (coefficient of determination, R^2 = 0.900 vs. 0.759). Implant size can be easily calculated by multiplying the healthy breast volume by 0.78 and adding 25 cc (ideal implant volume = healthy breast volume × 0.78 + 25 cc).

In order to develop a predictive model for satisfactory results after surgery, it is desirable to set the dependent variable as an ideal implant size rather than the inserted implant size. Most of the previous studies developed a prediction model based on the inserted implant. However, the inserted implant was not validated as an ideal implant size because postoperative evaluation was not performed in the previous studies. In the present study, we calculated the ideal implant size by correcting the inserted implant volume using the observed postoperative asymmetry in postoperative 3D surface imaging. Pohlmann et al. also calculated the ideal implant size by simply adding or subtracting the postoperative volume differences of both breasts [26]. However, 100 cc differences of the breast volume do not correspond to 100 cc differences of an implant. In the analysis of our data using inserted implant size and 3D breast volume, beta was 0.66 ($R2 = 88.0\%$, $p < 0.001$). The results suggested that a 100 cc difference corresponded to 66 cc of implant. Therefore, multiplying beta by the postoperative volume difference would be better for calculation of the ideal implant size.

One of significant findings of our study was that the beta values of the prediction model using 3D breast volume (0.78) and mastectomy specimen weight (0.84) were both less than 1. This result suggests that the ideal implant size should be smaller than the 3D breast volume or mastectomy specimen weight except when the breast size is small (<200 cc) (Figure 5). According to our prediction model, difference between ideal implant volume and 3-D volume of the healthy breast (or mastectomy weight) becomes larger as the breast size increases. This would be true because extent of oncologic resection is usually larger than the dimensions of the implant. In this case, the inserted implant makes central portions of the breast mound without covering peripheral area of the mastectomy defect. Similar with our study, Back et al. reported that long-term patient satisfaction was highest in a patient group whose implant volume to mastectomy specimen weight was 71.9% [10].

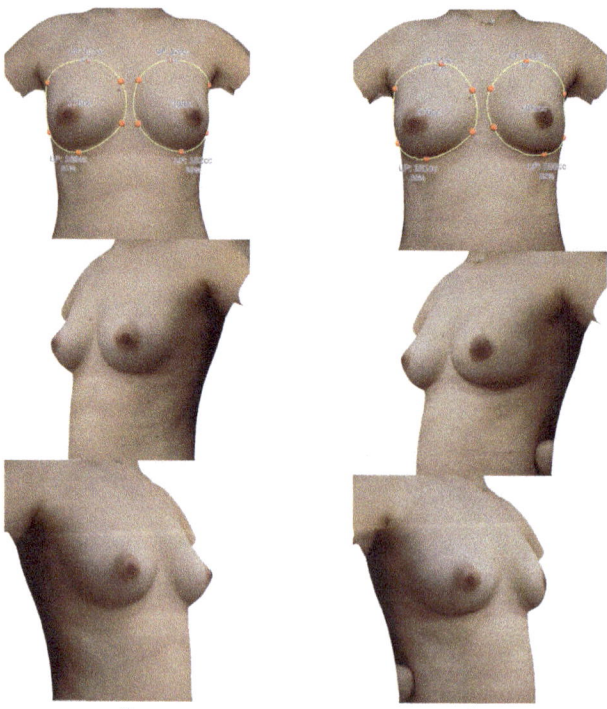

Figure 5. A case example of pre and postoperative 3-D volumes of the breasts. (**a**) Preoperative 3-D image. A 41-year-old woman with a diagnosis of left breast cancer. The volume of both breasts was 276 cc and 308 cc. The resected mastectomy specimen weight was 252 g and the inserted implant size was 275 cc. The operation was performed through periareolar incision, and the implant was inserted into the subpectoral plane. (**b**) Postoperative 3-D image. The volume of both breasts after three months of surgery was 276 cc and 302 cc. The volume on the reconstruction side was 9.4% larger.

Considering that our retrospective data set was relatively small, and the developed formulas have not been fully tested, the generalizability of these two formulas may requires more testing, especially in different populations. However, a relatively high coefficient of determination ($R^2 = 0.90$) could be obtained with statistical significance. The coefficient of determination in our prediction model ($R^2 = 0.90$) was higher than that of previous studies [11,13,26]. In terms of selection of the ideal implant in unilateral DTI breast reconstruction, implant volume is not the only factor to be considered for breast symmetry. Other various factors including breast width, breast height, projection, upper pole fullness, and degree of ptosis need to be considered together for the ideal implant volume for symmetry. Additionally, the size of the acellular dermal matrix influences the final volume of the reconstructed breast. The thickness and dimensions of the acellular dermal matrix should be considered, especially in prepectoral DTI, in which the implant is covered 360 degrees with the acellular dermal matrix.

5. Conclusions

Healthy breast volume measured by 3D surface imaging is a more accurate predictor than mastectomy specimen weight to estimate the implant volume for symmetry in DTI breast reconstruction. The estimation formula obtained in this study may assist in the selection of ideal implant size in unilateral DTI breast reconstruction.

Author Contributions: Conceptualization, K.-J.W.; Data curation, J.-H.K.; Formal analysis, J.-H.K. and J.-W.P.; Investigation, J.-W.P.; Methodology, J.-W.P. and K.-J.W.; Supervision, K.-J.W.; Writing—original draft, J.-H.K.; Writing—review and editing, J.-W.P. and K.-J.W. All authors have read and agreed to the published version of the manuscript.

Funding: This research received no external funding.

Conflicts of Interest: The authors declare no conflict of interest.

References

1. Azouz, V.; Lopez, S.; Wagner, D.S. Surgeon-Controlled Comparison of Direct-to-Implant and 2-Stage Tissue Expander-Implant Immediate Breast Reconstruction Outcomes. *Ann. Plast. Surg.* **2018**, *80*, 212–216. [CrossRef] [PubMed]
2. Kamali, P.; Koolen, P.G.L.; Ibrahim, A.M.S.; Paul, M.; Dikmans, R.E.; Schermerhorn, M.L.; Lee, B.T.; Lin, S.J. Analyzing Regional Differences over a 15-Year Trend of One-Stage versus Two-Stage Breast Reconstruction in 941,191 Postmastectomy Patients. *Plast. Reconstr. Surg.* **2016**, *138*, 1e–14e. [CrossRef] [PubMed]
3. Serrurier, L.C.J.; Rayne, S.; Venter, M.; Benn, C.-A. Direct-to-Implant Breast Reconstruction without the Use of an Acellular Dermal Matrix Is Cost Effective and Oncologically Safe. *Plast. Reconstr. Surg.* **2017**, *139*, 809–817. [CrossRef] [PubMed]
4. Chang, J.B.; Small, K.H.; Choi, M.; Karp, N.S. Three-Dimensional surface imaging in plastic surgery: Foundation, practical applications, and beyond. *Plast. Reconstr. Surg.* **2015**, *135*, 1295–1304. [CrossRef]
5. Galdino, G.M.; Nahabedian, M.; Chiaramonte, M.; Geng, J.Z.; Klatsky, S.; Manson, P. Clinical Applications of Three-Dimensional Photography in Breast Surgery. *Plast. Reconstr. Surg.* **2002**, *110*, 58–70. [CrossRef]
6. Tzou, C.H.; Artner, N.M.; Pona, I.; Hold, A.; Placheta, E.; Kropatsch, W.G.; Frey, M. Comparison of three-dimensional surface-imaging systems. *J. Plast. Reconstr. Aesthet. Surg.* **2014**, *67*, 489–497. [CrossRef]
7. Yip, J.M.; Mouratova, N.; Jeffery, R.M.; Veitch, D.E.; Woodman, R.J.; Dean, N.R. Accurate assessment of breast volume: A study comparing the volumetric gold standard (direct water displacement measurement of mastectomy specimen) with a 3D laser scanning technique. *Ann. Plast. Surg.* **2012**, *68*, 135–141. [CrossRef]
8. Georgii, J.; Eder, M.; Bürger, K.; Klotz, S.; Ferstl, F.; Kovács, L.; Westermann, R. A Computational Tool for Preoperative Breast Augmentation Planning in Aesthetic Plastic Surgery. *IEEE J. Biomed. Health Inform.* **2014**, *18*, 907–919. [CrossRef]
9. Henseler, H.; Hille-Betz, U.; Vogt, P. Validation of Subjective Estimates of Female Breast Volume and Comparison with Objective Methods. *Handchir. Mikrochir. Plast. Chir.* **2015**, *47*, 371–377. [CrossRef]
10. Baek, W.Y.; Byun, I.H.; Kim, Y.S.; Lew, D.H.; Jeong, J.; Roh, T.S. Patient Satisfaction with Implant Based Breast Reconstruction Associated with Implant Volume and Mastectomy Specimen Weight Ratio. *J. Breast Cancer* **2017**, *20*, 98–103. [CrossRef]

11. Georgiou, C.; Ihrai, T.; Chamorey, E.; Flipo, B.; Chignon-Sicard, B. A formula for implant volume choice in breast reconstruction after nipple sparing mastectomy. *Breast* **2012**, *21*, 781–782. [CrossRef]
12. Shia, W.; Yang, H.-J.; Wu, H.-K.; Lin, S.-L.; Lai, H.-W.; Huang, Y.-L.; Chen, D.-R. Implant volume estimation in direct-to-implant breast reconstruction after nipple-sparing mastectomy. *J. Surg. Res.* **2018**, *231*, 290–296. [CrossRef] [PubMed]
13. Wazir, U.; Chehade, H.E.H.; Choy, C.; Kasem, A.; Mokbel, K. A Study of the Relation Between Mastectomy Specimen Weight and Volume with Implant Size in Oncoplastic Reconstruction. *Vivo* **2019**, *33*, 125–132. [CrossRef] [PubMed]
14. Parmar, C.; West, M.; Pathak, S.; Nelson, J.; Martin, L. Weight versus volume in breast surgery: An observational study. *JRSM Short Rep.* **2011**, *2*, 1–5. [CrossRef] [PubMed]
15. Liu, C.; Luan, J.; Mu, L.; Ji, K. The Role of Three-Dimensional Scanning Technique in Evaluation of Breast Asymmetry in Breast Augmentation: A 100-Case Study. *Plast. Reconstr. Surg.* **2010**, *126*, 2125–2132. [CrossRef]
16. Chae, M.P.; Hunter-Smith, D.J.; Spychal, R.T.; Rozen, W.M. 3D volumetric analysis for planning breast reconstructive surgery. *Breast Cancer Res. Treat.* **2014**, *146*, 457–460. [CrossRef]
17. Erić, M.; Anderla, A.; Stefanović, D.; Drapšin, M. Breast volume estimation from systematic series of CT scans using the Cavalieri principle and 3D reconstruction. *Int. J. Surg.* **2014**, *12*, 912–917. [CrossRef]
18. Fujii, T.; Yamaguchi, S.; Yajima, R.; Tsutsumi, S.; Asao, T.; Kuwano, H. Accurate Assessment of Breast Volume by Computed Tomography Using Three-dimensional Imaging Device. *Am. Surg.* **2012**, *78*, 933–935. [CrossRef]
19. Kim, H.; Mun, G.-H.; Wiraatmadja, E.S.; Lim, S.-Y.; Pyon, J.-K.; Oh, K.S.; Lee, J.E.; Nam, S.J.; Lim, S.Y. Preoperative Magnetic Resonance Imaging-Based Breast Volumetry for Immediate Breast Reconstruction. *Aesthet. Plast. Surg.* **2015**, *39*, 369–376. [CrossRef]
20. Yoo, A.; Minn, K.W.; Jin, U.S. Magnetic Resonance Imaging-Based Volumetric Analysis and Its Relationship to Actual Breast Weight. *Arch. Plast. Surg.* **2013**, *40*, 203–208. [CrossRef]
21. Creasman, C.N.; Mordaunt, D.; Liolios, T.; Chiu, C.; Gabriel, A.; Maxwell, G.P. Four-Dimensional Breast Imaging, Part II: Clinical Implementation and Validation of a Computer Imaging System for Breast Augmentation Planning. *Aesthet. Surg. J.* **2011**, *31*, 925–938. [CrossRef] [PubMed]
22. Donfrancesco, A.; Montemurro, P.; Hedén, P. Three-Dimensional simulated images in breast augmentation surgery: An investigation of patients' satisfaction and the correlation between prediction and actual outcome. *Plast. Reconstr. Surg.* **2013**, *132*, 810–822. [CrossRef] [PubMed]
23. Gladilin, E.; Gabrielova, B.; Montemurro, P.; Hedén, P. Customized Planning of Augmentation Mammaplasty with Silicon Implants Using Three-Dimensional Optical Body Scans and Biomechanical Modeling of Soft Tissue Outcome. *Aesthet. Plast. Surg.* **2010**, *35*, 494–501. [CrossRef] [PubMed]
24. Vorstenbosch, J.; Islur, A. Correlation of Prediction and Actual Outcome of Three-Dimensional Simulation in Breast Augmentation Using a Cloud-Based Program. *Aesthet. Plast. Surg.* **2017**, *133*, 481–490. [CrossRef]
25. Roostaeian, J.; Adams, W.P., Jr. Three-Dimensional Imaging for Breast Augmentation: Is This Technology Providing Accurate Simulations? *Aesthet. Surg. J.* **2014**, *34*, 857–875. [CrossRef]
26. Pöhlmann, S.T.L.; Harkness, E.; Taylor, C.J.; Gandhi, A.; Astley, S.M. Preoperative implant selection for unilateral breast reconstruction using 3D imaging with the Microsoft Kinect sensor. *J. Plast. Reconstr. Aesthet. Surg.* **2017**, *70*, 1059–1067. [CrossRef]

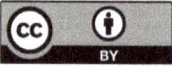

© 2020 by the authors. Licensee MDPI, Basel, Switzerland. This article is an open access article distributed under the terms and conditions of the Creative Commons Attribution (CC BY) license (http://creativecommons.org/licenses/by/4.0/).

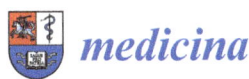

Article

Intraoperative Intercostal Nerve Block for Postoperative Pain Control in Pre-Pectoral versus Subpectoral Direct-To-Implant Breast Reconstruction: A Retrospective Study

Jin-Woo Park, Jeong Hoon Kim and Kyong-Je Woo *

Department of Plastic and Reconstructive Surgery, Ewha Womans University Mokdong Hospital, College of Medicine, Ewha Womans University, Seoul 07985, Korea; burnscar@naver.com (J.-W.P.); kimsbrothers@hanmail.net (J.H.K.)
* Correspondence: economywoo@gmail.com

Received: 24 May 2020; Accepted: 27 June 2020; Published: 30 June 2020

Abstract: *Background and Objectives:* Patients undergoing mastectomy and implant-based breast reconstruction have significant acute postsurgical pain. The purpose of this study was to examine the efficacy of intercostal nerve blocks (ICNBs) for reducing pain after direct-to-implant (DTI) breast reconstruction. *Materials and Methods:* Between January 2019 and March 2020, patients who underwent immediate DTI breast reconstruction were included in this study. The patients were divided into the ICNB or control group. In the ICNB group, 4 cc of 0.2% ropivacaine was injected intraoperatively to the second, third, fourth, and fifth intercostal spaces just before implant insertion. The daily average and maximum visual analogue scale (VAS) scores were recorded by the patient from operative day to postoperative day (POD) seven. Pain scores were compared between the ICNB and control groups and analyzed according to the insertion plane of implants. *Results:* A total of 67 patients with a mean age of 47.9 years were included; 31 patients received ICNBs and 36 patients did not receive ICNBs. There were no complications related to ICNBs reported. The ICNB group showed a significantly lower median with an average VAS score on the operative day (4 versus 6, $p = 0.047$), lower maximum VAS scores on the operative day (5 versus 7.5, $p = 0.030$), and POD 1 (4 versus 6, $p = 0.030$) as compared with the control group. Among patients who underwent subpectoral reconstruction, the ICNB group showed a significantly lower median with an average VAS score on the operative day (4 versus 7, $p = 0.005$), lower maximum VAS scores on the operative day (4.5 versus 8, $p = 0.004$), and POD 1 (4 versus 6, $p = 0.009$), whereas no significant differences were observed among those who underwent pre-pectoral reconstruction. *Conclusions:* Intraoperative ICNBs can effectively reduce immediate postoperative pain in subpectoral DTI breast reconstruction; however, it may not be effective in pre-pectoral DTI reconstruction.

Keywords: intercostal nerve block; postoperative pain; pain control; direct-to-implant breast reconstruction; prosthesis; implant

---

1. Introduction

The adequate management of immediate postoperative pain after breast surgery is important for improving patients' well-being in the immediate postoperative period and for reducing pain-induced restriction of movement predisposing patients to poor recovery [1]. Inadequate management of pain in the immediate postoperative period affects patients' life quality and can also have severe consequences such as chronic postoperative pain [2–5]. The incidence of chronic postoperative pain after mastectomy and breast reconstruction has been reported in up to 50% of patients [6–8].

The management of immediate postoperative pain includes the use of intravenous analgesics, botulinum toxin, glucocorticoids, muscle relaxers, nonsteroidal agents, indwelling pain catheters, paravertebral nerve blocks, and intercostal nerve blocks (ICNBs) [1,4]. Among them, ICNBs were introduced in mastectomy by McCann [9] as an adjunctive to general anesthesia, and the use of ICNBs has been reported to be a safe and effective method to manage immediate postoperative pain in patients undergoing tissue expander reconstruction [1] and augmentation mammoplasty [10,11]. ICNBs can be performed in breast reconstruction under the direct vision of the intercostal spaces intraoperatively by the operator without an anesthesiologist [1].

Direct-to-implant (DTI) breast reconstruction is one of the most recent advances in breast reconstruction and is currently gaining popularity [12–14] due to its oncologic safety, cost effectiveness, and aesthetic outcome [15–18]. Several studies have investigated the techniques and surgical and aesthetic outcomes of DTI breast reconstruction; however, limited studies have examined the use of intraoperative ICNBs with a local anesthetic for patients undergoing DTI breast reconstruction [1]. Particularly, there have been no studies that have evaluated the differences in the natural course and management of pain according to the insertion plane of implants. The main objective of the current study was to evaluate the efficacy of intraoperative nerve blocks using ropivacaine for postoperative pain after DTI breast reconstruction. The secondary objective was to compare pain scores between pre-pectoral and subpectoral DTI breast reconstruction.

2. Materials and Methods

2.1. Patient Cohort

The study was conducted in accordance with the Declaration of Helsinki, and the protocol was approved by the institutional review board of Ewha Womans University Mokdong Hospital (no. 2020-05-01). Consecutive patients who underwent immediate unilateral DTI reconstruction with an acellular dermal matrix at our institution between January 2019 and March 2020 were retrospectively reviewed. Patients who were given intravenous patient-controlled analgesia (IV PCA) postoperatively were included. Patients who had a previous breast procedure, including breast-conserving surgery for previous malignancy, augmentation mammoplasty, mastopexy, and reduction mammoplasty, and a history of radiation therapy were excluded from this study. A modified Charlson comorbidity index was calculated as a summation of the overall extent of comorbidities for each patient [19,20]. Three experienced oncologic surgeons with over 10 years of experience performed the mastectomies, and the senior author (K.-J.W.) performed all reconstruction procedures.

2.2. Surgical Technique

Single-stage breast reconstruction with silicone gel implants was performed in all nipple-sparing mastectomy (NSM) cases and skin-sparing mastectomy (SSM) cases with minimal skin flap excisions. Under a general anesthesia, IV fentanyl (Hana Pharm Co., Ltd., Seoul, Korea) was routinely administered with a dose of 3 µg per kg of the patient's body weight. For patients who could not afford a large acellular dermal matrix, had a thin mastectomy skin flap (which can cause significant rippling), or had compromised mastectomy skin flap perfusion, the implant was placed in the subpectoral space. An acellular dermal matrix (human cadaveric) was used for inferior and lateral support and implant coverage. Otherwise, implants were placed in pre-pectoral spaces and draped with a 16 × 16 cm or 18 × 18 cm acellular dermal matrix. For patients receiving nerve blocks, 4 cc of 0.2% ropivacaine (Mitsubishi Tanabe Pharma Korea Co., Ltd., Seoul, Korea) was injected into each intercostal space from T2 to T5 just before the placement of the implant. A syringe (10 cc) was connected to a 23-gauge butterfly needle to check and maintain the penetration depth during injection. The needle was angled 15° cephalad, and the penetration depth was 5 mm, which was marked by a sterile tape on the needle to achieve a consistent depth of injection as previously described [21]. Injections were given after a surgeon confirmed that neither blood nor air was aspirated. Injection sites were the most lateral portion of accessible 2nd to 5th intercostal spaces near the mid to anterior axillary line [1,4]. After the placement of the implant, two closed suction drains were placed in the subpectoral and pre-pectoral spaces for subpectoral reconstruction and in the upper and lower pole of the pre-pectoral spaces for pre-pectoral reconstruction. Drains were removed when the drainage amount was less than 30 mL over 24 h for two consecutive days. Patients were discharged after all of the surgical drains were removed. Prophylactic antibiotics were administrated until drain removal.

After the surgery, fentanyl was administered intravenously according to the patient's vital signs or complaint of pain in the post-anesthesia care unit (PACU). An IV PCA device administering fentanyl and ramosetron (Daiichi Sankyo Korea Co., Ltd., Seoul, Korea) was routinely used after surgery. The IV PCA started with a total volume of 60 mL consisting of 10–12 µg fentanyl per kg of the patient's body weight and was continuously infused at a rate of 0.5 mL/h. The device was set to deliver 0.5 mL boluses whenever the patient pressed the designated button. Patients were encouraged to press the button whenever they felt pain. The IV PCA device was removed at 48 h postoperatively, and the remaining dose was measured. After the IV PCA device was removed, aceclofenac (100 mg) was administered orally twice daily for pain control. When the patient required additional analgesia, pain control was augmented using IV acetaminophen, IV ketorolac, or oral acetaminophen. For comparison, pain medications were converted to morphine equivalents to calculate the total usage of pain medication. Morphine equivalents administered in the PACU and after the PACU were analyzed.

Patients were educated about visual analogue scale (VAS) scores on the day before the surgery. The daily average and maximum VAS scores were recorded by the patient using a self-recording VAS score sheet, which was given to the patient at the time of patient education. A VAS score of 5 was defined as the degree of pain at which the patient found it difficult to sleep or rest without additional pain control, and a VAS score of 10 was defined as pain as severe as death. Pain degree was recorded from the operative day to postoperative day 7. The VAS score sheets were collected after postoperative day 7 and analyzed. If patients were discharged earlier than postoperative day 7, an oral pain medication was prescribed, and patients were asked to complete the self-recording VAS score sheet and the sheets were retrieved at the first visit to the outpatient clinic. All patients, except two, patients were discharged after 7 postoperative days.

2.3. Analysis

Data obtained from the chart review included postoperative PCA usage and patient-reported VAS pain scores from the day of operation to postoperative day 7. The daily average and maximum VAS scores were compared between the pre-pectoral reconstruction and subpectoral reconstruction groups for patients who did not receive ICNBs to analyze the natural course of postoperative pain according to the insertion plane of implants. To evaluate the effect of ICNBs, the daily average and maximum VAS scores were compared between the ICNB and control groups for all patients. The subgroup analyses were performed on the insertion plane of implants to evaluate the difference in the effect of ICNBs between patients who underwent subpectoral reconstruction and those who underwent pre-pectoral reconstruction.

The mean with standard deviation or median with interquartile range were used to summarize continuous variables based on the distribution of the data, and the frequency and proportion were used to describe categorical variables. Shapiro–Wilk tests were conducted to test normal distribution. The clinical and operative variables were compared between the groups using two-sample t-test or Mann–Whitney U test for continuous variables and the Chi-squared test or Fisher's exact test for categorical variables. The statistical significance was determined by $p < 0.05$. All analyses were performed using SPSS version 23.0 (SPSS Inc., Chicago, IL, USA).

3. Results

Among 78 patients who underwent DTI breast reconstruction after NSM or SSM in the study period, 67 patients met the inclusion criteria and were included in this study. A total of 11 patients were excluded as they did not use IV PCA or discontinued using it before 48 h postoperatively due to side effects. There were no immediate nerve block-related complications observed in patients who received intraoperative ICNBs. A total of 33 patients (49.3%) underwent DTI breast reconstruction with pre-pectoral placement of the implant, and the remaining 34 patients (50.7%) had subpectoral implant placement. The mean patient age was 47.91 ± 8.06 years, and the mean body mass index (BMI) was 22.63 ± 2.63 kg/m^2. There were no significant differences between the pre-pectoral and subpectoral reconstruction groups in age, BMI, Charlson comorbidity index score, smoking history, previous chemotherapy, mastectomy type, axillary lymph node management, and morphine equivalents. The mastectomy weight was significantly higher in the subpectoral group than in the pre-pectoral group (312.3 g versus 236.4 g, $p = 0.019$); however, the implant volume was not significantly different between the two groups (325.7 mL versus 285.9 mL, $p = 0.103$) (Table 1).

Table 1. Clinical and surgical characteristics.

	Overall Patients (n = 67)	Pre-Pectoral (n = 33)	Subpectoral (n = 34)	p
Age, mean ± SD, yr	47.91 ± 8.06	47.12 ± 8.37	48.68 ± 7.80	0.434 *
BMI, mean ± SD, kg/m^2	22.63 ± 2.63	22.34 ± 2.63	22.92 ± 2.64	0.377 *
Charlson comorbidity index, median (IQR), score	2 (2–3)	2 (2–3)	2 (2–3)	0.911 †
Smoking history, n (%)	3 (4.1)	3 (9.1)	0	0.114 §
Preoperative chemotherapy, n (%)	6 (9.0)	3 (9.1)	3 (8.8)	>0.999 §
Mastectomy type, n (%)				0.673 §
Nipple-sparing	61 (91.0)	31 (93.9)	30 (88.2)	
Skin-sparing	6 (9.0)	2 (6.1)	4 (11.8)	
Mastectomy weight, mean ± SD, g	274.9 ± 133.6	236.4 ± 100.7	312.3 ± 151.5	0.019 *
Implant volume, mean ± SD, mL	306.1 ± 99.8	285.9 ± 85.0	325.7 ± 110.0	0.103 *
Axillary lymph node management, n (%)				0.701 ‡
None	0	0	0	
SLNB	56 (83.6)	27 (81.8)	29 (85.3)	
ALND	11 (16.4)	6 (18.2)	5 (14.7)	
Morphine equivalents, median (IQR), mg				
PACU	3 (0–5)	5 (3–5)	3 (0–5)	0.474 †
After the PACU	189.5 (184.5–198.75)	189.5 (184.5–198)	191.5 (184.5–199)	0.339 †

SD, standard deviation; BMI, body mass index; IQR, interquartile range; SLNB, sentinel lymph node biopsy; ALND, axillary lymph node dissection; PACU, post-anesthesia care unit. * p value obtained in 2-sampled t-test. † p values obtained in Mann–Whitney U test. ‡ p value obtained in Chi-squared test. § p values obtained in Fisher's exact test.

The comparison of VAS scores between the pre-pectoral and subpectoral reconstruction groups for patients who did not receive ICNBs is shown in Table 2. On the operative day, the subpectoral reconstruction group showed a higher median with an average VAS score (7 versus 6, $p = 0.062$) with marginal significance. The maximum VAS score (8 versus 6.5, $p = 0.108$) was higher on the operative day; however, the difference did not reach statistical significance. The average and maximum VAS scores were also higher among patients who underwent subpectoral reconstruction than among those who underwent pre-pectoral reconstruction from postoperative day one to day seven; however, the difference was not statistically significant.

Table 2. Comparison of postoperative visual analogue scale (VAS) scores between pre-pectoral and subpectoral reconstructions for patients who did not undergo intercostal nerve block.

	Pre-Pectoral Reconstruction	Subpectoral Reconstruction	p
Average VAS, median (IQR), score			
Operative day	6 (3–6.75)	7 (5–8)	0.062 *
POD 1	4 (3–5)	5 (3.25–6.75)	0.122 †
POD 2	3.5 (2–4)	4 (3–5)	0.268 †
POD 3	2.5 (2–4)	3 (2–4.75)	0.448 †
POD 4	2 (2–3)	3 (2–4)	0.293 †
POD 5	2 (1–2.75)	2 (2–3)	0.623 †
POD 6	2 (0.25–2)	2 (1–2)	0.656 †
POD 7	1.5 (0–2)	2 (1–2)	0.571 †
Maximum VAS, median (IQR), score			
Operative day	6.5 (4–8)	8 (6–10)	0.108 †
POD 1	5 (4–6)	6 (4–8)	0.114 †
POD 2	4 (3–6)	4 (4–6)	0.692 †
POD 3	3.5 (2–4.75)	4 (2–5.75)	0.937 †
POD 4	3 (2–4)	4 (2–4)	0.660 †
POD 5	3 (2–4)	2 (2–3.75)	0.840 †
POD 6	2 (2–2)	2 (2–3)	0.577 †
POD 7	2 (1–2.75)	2 (1.25–3)	0.720 †

VAS, visual analogue scale; IQR, interquartile range; POD, postoperative day. * p value obtained in 2-sampled t-test.
† p values obtained in Mann–Whitney U test.

3.1. Comparison of Pain Scores between the ICNB and Control Groups

Among the selected 67 patients, 31 patients were included in the ICNB group, and the remaining 36 patients were included in the control group. Table 3 shows the comparison of clinical and surgical characteristics between the ICNB and control groups. There were no significant differences between the two groups in age, BMI, Charlson comorbidity index score, smoking history, previous chemotherapy, mastectomy type, mastectomy weight, implant volume, axillary lymph node management, and morphine equivalents. In the comparison of daily VAS scores between the ICNB and control groups, the median of average (4 versus 6, $p = 0.047$) and maximum (5 versus 7.5, $p = 0.030$) VAS scores on the operative day and maximum (4 versus 6, $p = 0.030$) VAS score on postoperative day one were significantly lower in the ICNB group than in the control group (Table 4).

3.2. Subpectoral Reconstruction

Among 34 patients who underwent subpectoral reconstruction, 16 patients were included in the ICNB group, and 18 patients were included in the control group. There were no significant differences between the ICNB and control groups in age, BMI, Charlson comorbidity index score, smoking history, previous chemotherapy, mastectomy type, mastectomy weight, implant volume, axillary lymph node management, and morphine equivalents (Table 5). Figure 1 shows the significant differences in the average and maximum VAS scores on the operative day and maximum VAS score on postoperative day one between the ICNB and control groups. On the operative day, the median of the average (4 versus 7, $p = 0.005$) and maximum (4.5 versus 8, $p = 0.004$) VAS scores were significantly lower in the ICNB group than in the control group. On postoperative day one, the median of the average VAS score was lower in the ICNB group than in the control group with marginal significance (3.5 versus 5, $p = 0.060$), and the maximum VAS score was significantly lower in the ICNB group than in the control group (4 versus 6, $p = 0.009$).

Table 3. Comparison of clinical and surgical characteristics between the intercostal nerve block (ICNB) and control groups in overall patients.

	ICNB Group (n = 31)	Control Group (n = 36)	p
Age, mean ± SD, yr	48.26 ± 7.81	47.61 ± 8.37	0.746 *
BMI, mean ± SD, kg/m^2	22.66 ± 2.63	22.62 ± 2.67	0.953 *
Charlson comorbidity index, median (IQR), score	2 (2–3)	2 (2–3)	0.928 †
Smoking history, n (%)	1 (3.2)	2 (5.6)	>0.999 §
Preoperative chemotherapy, n (%)	3 (9.7)	3 (8.3)	>0.999 §
Mastectomy type, n (%)			0.404 §
Nipple-sparing	27 (87.1)	34 (94.4)	
Skin-sparing	4 (12.9)	2 (5.6)	
Mastectomy weight, mean ± SD, g	251.6 ± 124.1	295.0 ± 139.9	0.187 *
Implant volume, mean ± SD, mL	282.6 ± 81.7	326.4 ± 110.2	0.073 *
Axillary lymph node management, n (%)			0.953 ‡
None	0	0	
SLNB	26 (83.9)	30 (83.3)	
ALND	5 (16.1)	6 (16.7)	
Morphine equivalents, median (IQR), mg			
PACU	5 (3–5)	3 (0–5)	0.474 †
After the PACU	189.5 (180.5–198.75)	191.5 (184.95–198)	0.339 †

ICNB, intercostal nerve block; SD, standard deviation; BMI, body mass index; IQR, interquartile range; SLNB, sentinel lymph node biopsy; ALND, axillary lymph node dissection; PACU, post-anesthesia care unit. * p value obtained in 2-sampled t-test. † p values obtained in Mann–Whitney U test. ‡ p value obtained in Chi-squared test. § p values obtained in Fisher's exact test.

Table 4. Comparison of postoperative VAS scores between the ICNB and control groups in overall patients.

	ICNB Group	Control Group	p
Average VAS, median (IQR), score			
Operative day	4 (3.5–6)	6 (4–8)	0.047 *
POD 1	4 (2–4.5)	4 (3–6)	0.104 †
POD 2	3 (2–4)	4 (2–4.25)	0.365 *
POD 3	2 (1–4)	3 (2–4)	0.487 †
POD 4	2 (1–3)	2.5 (2–4)	0.108 †
POD 5	2 (1–3)	2 (1–3)	0.688 †
POD 6	1 (1–2)	2 (0.75–2)	0.190 †
POD 7	1 (0.5–2)	2 (0–2)	0.117 †
Maximum VAS, median (IQR), score			
Operative day	5 (4–8)	7.5 (5–8)	0.030 †
POD 1	4 (3–5.5)	6 (4–7.25)	0.030 *
POD 2	4 (2–4.5)	4 (3–6)	0.137 †
POD 3	2 (2–4)	4 (2–5.25)	0.301 †
POD 4	2 (2–3.5)	3 (2–4)	0.068 †
POD 5	2 (1–3)	2 (2–4)	0.272 †
POD 6	2 (1–2)	2 (2–3)	0.190 †
POD 7	2 (0.5–2)	2 (1–3)	0.117 †

ICNB, intercostal nerve block; VAS, visual analogue scale; IQR, interquartile range. * p value obtained in 2-sampled t-test. † p values obtained in Mann–Whitney U test.

3.3. Pre-Pectoral Reconstruction

Among 33 patients who underwent pre-pectoral reconstruction, 15 patients were included in the ICNB group, and 18 patients were included in the control group. There were no significant differences between the ICNB and control groups in age, BMI, Charlson comorbidity index score, smoking history, previous chemotherapy, mastectomy type, mastectomy weight, implant volume, axillary lymph node management, and morphine equivalents (Table 6). Figure 2 compares the postoperative average and maximum VAS scores between the ICNB and control groups. Both the average and maximum VAS scores were decreased with each successive postoperative day. On the operative day, the median of the average VAS score was 5 in the ICNB group and 6 in the control group ($p = 0.891$), and the maximum VAS score was 5 in the ICNB group and 6 in the control group ($p = 0.782$). On postoperative day one, the median of the average VAS score was 4 in the ICNB group and 4 in the control group ($p = 0.821$), and the maximum VAS score was 5 in the ICNB group and 5 in the control group ($p = 0.589$). There were no significant differences in VAS scores between the ICNB and control groups from the operative day to postoperative day seven.

Table 5. Comparison of clinical and surgical characteristics between the ICNB and control groups for patients who underwent subpectoral reconstruction.

	ICNB Group (n = 16)	Control Group (n = 18)	p
Age, mean ± SD, yr	46.69 ± 7.56	47.78 ± 8.11	0.484 *
BMI, mean ± SD, kg/m^2	23.1 ± 2.56	22.75 ± 2.77	0.696 *
Charlson comorbidity index, median (IQR), score	2 (2–4)	2 (2e3)	0.874 †
Smoking history, n (%)	0	0	-
Preoperative chemotherapy, n (%)	2 (12.5)	1 (5.6)	0.591 ‡
Mastectomy type, n (%)			>0.999 ‡
Nipple-sparing	15 (93.8)	16 (88.9)	
Skin-sparing	1 (6.3)	2 (11.1)	
Mastectomy weight, mean ± SD, g	277.9 ± 136.8	342.9 ± 160.9	0.217 *
Implant volume, mean ± SD, mL	292.2 ± 92.0	355.6 ± 118.4	0.094 *
Axillary lymph node management, n (%)			>0.999 ‡
None	0	0	
SLNB	14 (87.5)	15 (83.3)	
ALND	2 (12.5)	3 (16.7)	
Morphine equivalents, median (IQR), mg			
PACU	3 (0–5)	4 (0–5)	0.880 †
After the PACU	189.5 (181–196.5)	191.5 (185.75–204.3)	0.115 †

ICNB, intercostal nerve block; SD, standard deviation; BMI, body mass index; IQR, interquartile range; SLNB, sentinel lymph node biopsy; ALND, axillary lymph node dissection; PACU, post-anesthesia care unit. * p value obtained in 2-sampled t-test. † p values obtained in Mann–Whitney U test. ‡ p values obtained in Fisher's exact test.

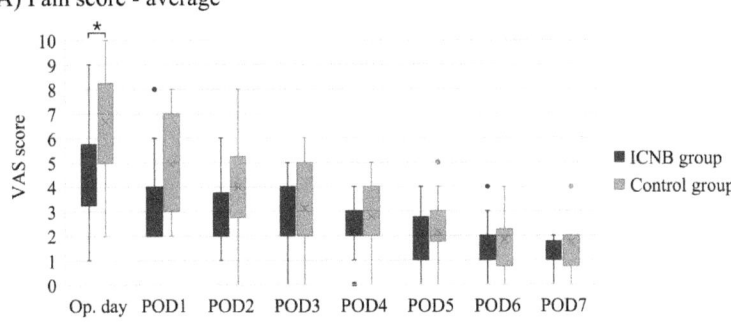

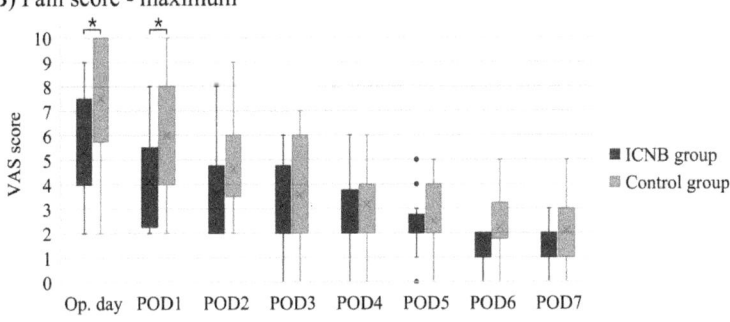

Figure 1. Comparison of postoperative daily average (**A**) and maximum (**B**) visual analogue scale (VAS) pain scores between the intercostal nerve block (ICNB) and control groups for patients who underwent subpectoral direct-to-implant (DTI) breast reconstruction. POD, postoperative day. * means that the differences are statistically significant; • indicates outliers in the box-and-whisker plots.

Table 6. Comparison of clinical and surgical characteristics between ICNB and control groups for patients who underwent pre-pectoral reconstruction.

	ICNB Group (n = 15)	Control Group (n = 18)	p
Age, mean ± SD, yr	46.73 ± 8.04	47.44 ± 8.85	0.812 *
BMI, mean ± SD, kg/m²	22.17 ± 2.70	22.49 ± 2.65	0.738 *
Charlson comorbidity index score, median (IQR), score	2 (2–3)	2 (2–3.75)	0.997 †
Smoking history, n (%)	1 (6.7)	2 (11.1)	>0.999 ‡
Preoperative chemotherapy, n (%)	1 (6.7)	2 (11.1)	>0.999 ‡
Mastectomy type, n (%)			>0.999 ‡
Nipple-sparing	13 (86.7)	18 (100.0)	
Skin-sparing	2 (13.3)	0	
Mastectomy weight, mean ± SD, g	223.5 ± 106.2	247.1 ± 97.7	0.532 *
Implant volume, mean ± SD, mL	272.3 ± 70.8	297.2 ± 95.8	0.411 *
Axillary lymph node management, n (%)			>0.999 ‡
None	0	0	
SLNB	12 (80.0)	15 (83.3)	
ALND	3 (20.0)	3 (16.7)	
Morphine equivalents, median (IQR), mg			
PACU	3 (0–5)	5 (3–5)	0.901 †
After the PACU	189.5 (185.9–202)	189.5 (184.65–196)	0.714 †

ICNB, intercostal nerve block; SD, standard deviation; BMI, body mass index; IQR, interquartile range; SLNB, sentinel lymph node biopsy; ALND, axillary lymph node dissection; PACU, post-anesthesia care unit. * p value obtained in 2-sampled t-test. † p values obtained in Mann–Whitney U test. ‡ p values obtained in Fisher's exact test.

A) Pain score - average

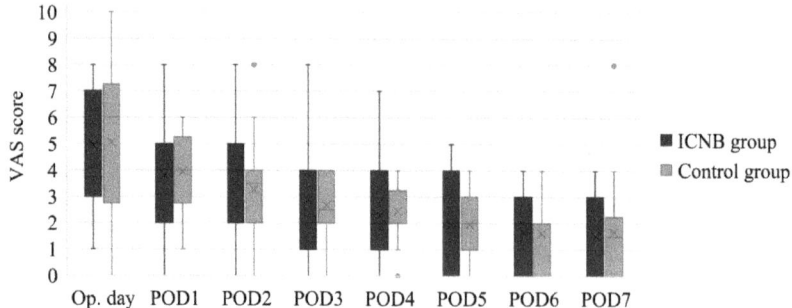

B) Pain score - maximum

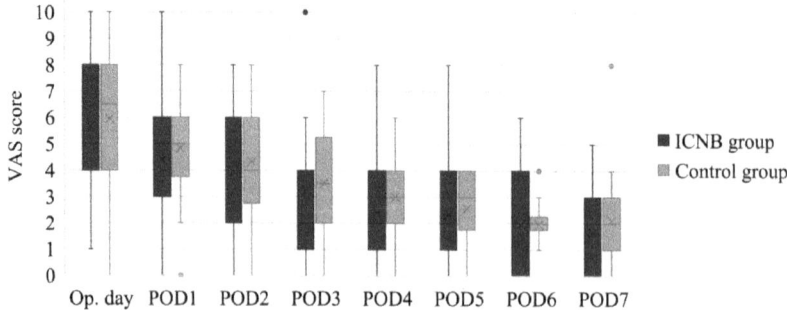

Figure 2. Comparison of postoperative daily average (A) and maximum (B) VAS pain scores between the ICNB and control groups for patients who underwent pre-pectoral DTI breast reconstruction. • indicates outliers in the box-and-whisker plots.

4. Discussion

We evaluated the effect of intraoperative ICNBs on postoperative pain after DTI breast reconstruction in cases of NSM or SSM using VAS scores and demonstrated that ICNBs significantly reduced postoperative pain in subpectoral DTI reconstruction during the immediate postoperative period; however, there were no significant differences in VAS scores observed between the ICNB and control groups in pre-pectoral reconstruction. Among patients who underwent subpectoral DTI reconstruction, the average VAS score was significantly decreased on the operative day and the maximum VAS score was significantly decreased on the operative day and postoperative day one in the ICNB group. There were no immediate complications related to the nerve block procedure observed.

Several studies have evaluated the effect of ICNBs on postoperative pain after implant-based breast reconstruction. However, to the best of our knowledge, no studies have examined the differences between subpectoral and pre-pectoral reconstructions. Butz et al. [22] evaluated the effect of intraoperative injection of liposomal bupivacaine in immediate breast reconstruction with the subpectoral placement of a tissue expander and demonstrated that the length of hospital stay and postoperative VAS pain scores were significantly lower in the liposomal bupivacaine group as compared with the pain pump and control groups. On the one hand, Shah et al. [1] assessed the effect of intraoperative administration of bupivacaine in subpectoral DTI reconstruction and found that the consumption of pain medication and length of hospital stay were significantly decreased among patients receiving ICNBs as compared with those who did not. On the other hand, Lanier et al. [4] compared the quality of recovery scores, pain scores, and opioid consumption between the ICNB and placebo groups for patients undergoing immediate breast reconstruction with subpectoral placement of a tissue expander and observed no significant differences between the two groups.

Intercostal nerves arise from the anterior divisions of the thoracic spinal nerves from T1 to T11 [23]. Intercostal nerves supply the sensory innervation for the back, trunk, and upper abdomen as well as the muscular innervation for the intercostal muscles. In addition to distribution to the muscle and skin, branches of the intercostal nerves supply the parietal pleura, mammary glands, and periosteum of the ribs [23,24]. The lateral cutaneous branches are derived from the intercostal nerves around midway between the vertebrae and sternum, which give cutaneous information from the skin of the lateral thoracic wall. The anterior cutaneous branches are the terminal branches of the intercostal nerves, which supply the skin of the anterior thoracic wall. In this study, the exact reason for the superior pain control using ICNBs in subpectoral reconstruction as compared with pre-pectoral reconstruction remains unclear; however, we hypothesized that sensory block of the periosteum could have contributed to the increased effectiveness of ICNBs in subpectoral reconstruction as compared with pre-pectoral reconstruction. The periosteum is highly vascularized and highly innervated by both sympathetic and pain-sensitive fibers [25,26], and mechanical destruction or distortion can cause significant pain [27]. ICNB has been demonstrated to be effective in the management of bone pain [28], which was derived from damage of the periosteum [29]. In subpectoral reconstruction, the periosteum can be easily damaged during the dissection of the subpectoral space and hemostasis of the well-vascularized periosteum. In addition, direct compression of the periosteum by the subpectoral placement of the implant can irritate or distort the periosteum and cause pain. The pain derived from the periosteum of the ribs might be managed by ICNBs. To block collateral branches to the periosteum, the nerve trunk should be targeted rather than cutaneous branches when performing ICNBs.

The findings of previous studies support our hypothesis that sensory block of the periosteum can contribute to the effectiveness of ICNBs in subpectoral breast reconstruction. A study by Lanier et al. [4] revealed that intraoperative nerve blocks failed to improve pain scores in subpectoral tissue expander reconstruction. They performed nerve blocks by injecting bupivacaine and dexamethasone around the anterior and lateral cutaneous branches of the intercostal nerves. In addition, Shah et al. [1] targeted the intercostal nerve trunk in their case series involving subpectoral DTI breast reconstruction and showed a significant decrease in the consumption of pain medication and length of hospital stay following

ICNBs. We believe that sensory block of the periosteum by targeting the intercostal nerve trunk is an essential part of ICNBs in subpectoral breast reconstruction.

When VAS scores were compared among patients who did not receive ICNBs, scores in the immediate postoperative period were lower in the pre-pectoral reconstruction group than in the subpectoral reconstruction group. Although the difference did not reach statistical significance, the average VAS score on the operative day was lower in the pre-pectoral reconstruction group with borderline significance (6 versus 7, $p = 0.062$). Previous studies have shown controversial results; some studies reported significantly lower pain scores in pre-pectoral reconstruction than in subpectoral reconstruction [30–32], whereas other studies reported that the pain scores were not significantly different [33,34]. Further meta-analysis should be conducted to confirm the significantly lower postoperative pain in pre-pectoral reconstruction as compared with subpectoral reconstruction.

ICNBs could be recommended for patients undergoing subpectoral DTI breast reconstruction for three reasons. First, according to the results of this study, a rapid reduction in VAS pain scores was observed with each successive postoperative day in the immediate postoperative period after subpectoral DTI breast reconstruction. The medians of average VAS scores were 7 (5–8), 5 (3.25–6.75), and 4 (3–5) on the operative day, postoperative day one, and postoperative day two, respectively, among patients who did not receive ICNBs. ICNBs can reduce immediate postoperative pain, and pain after the immediate postoperative period can be effectively managed with conventional analgesia. Secondly, ICNBs have minimal risk for procedure-related complications. Complications after ICNBs include pneumothorax, systemic toxic reactions to local anesthetics, abscess formation, and neuritis [10]. Among them, pneumothorax can be the most severe complication; however, its incidence after ICNBs is rare and has been reported as 0.073–4% [35–37]. Moore et al. [35] reported that therapeutic intervention was not required for pneumothorax in their analysis of 10,941 ICNB cases, and severe systemic toxic reactions did not occur. Third, ICNBs can be easily performed by the operating surgeon and do not require an anesthesiologist and the additional positioning of the patient, whereas paravertebral blocks are administered preoperatively by an anesthesiologist while the patient is awake, which can cause significant discomfort to the patient [1]. Moreover, paravertebral blocks bear certain risks according to the neuroaxial location [38]. In terms of the efficacy of the nerve block procedures, ICNB has been demonstrated to be effective in breast surgeries and combined blockade of the pectoral nerves, the intercostobrachial, intercostals III–IV–V–VI, and the long thoracic nerve (Pecs II block) was suggested to be more effective than paravertebral blocks in breast surgeries [39,40]. Nerve block targets for effective pain control in breast surgeries could be a good subject for further research.

The current study had some limitations. First, in the subgroup analysis, the average postoperative VAS score was higher in the subpectoral reconstruction group than in the pre-pectoral reconstruction group for patients who did not receive ICNBs at early postoperative days; however, the difference did not reach statistical significance. A possible explanation for the lack of statistical significance is the small number of patients. Further large-scale studies would be necessary to compare the postoperative pain scores between the subpectoral and pre-pectoral reconstruction groups. Secondly, the daily dose of pain medication could not be assessed because the remaining dose of IV PCA was measured after the IV PCA device was removed. The daily dose of pain medication could be higher in the subpectoral reconstruction than in the pre-pectoral reconstruction because the average and maximum VAS scores were significantly higher in the subpectoral reconstruction in the immediate postoperative period, but the difference of the daily dose of pain medication was not assessed. Last, the groups could be skewed due to the retrospective study design. Taking into consideration the results of this study, a double-blind randomized clinical trial should be performed to confirm the results of this study.

5. Conclusions

ICNBs could be a safe and effective method for the pain control of patients undergoing subpectoral DTI breast reconstruction. Intraoperative ICNBs can effectively reduce immediate postoperative pain in subpectoral DTI breast reconstruction; however, it may not be effective in pre-pectoral DTI reconstruction. The nerve trunk should be targeted to block collateral branches to the periosteum of the ribs when performing ICNBs.

Author Contributions: Conceptualization, K.-J.W.; Data curation, J.H.K.; Formal analysis, J.-W.P. and J.H.K.; Investigation, J.-W.P.; Methodology, J.-W.P. and K.-J.W.; Supervision, K.-J.W.; Writing—original draft, J.-W.P. and J.H.K.; Writing—review and editing, J.-W.P. and K.-J.W. All authors have read and agreed to the published version of the manuscript.

Funding: This research received no external funding.

Conflicts of Interest: The authors declare no conflict of interest.

References

1. Shah, A.; Rowlands, M.; Krishnan, N.; Patel, A.; Ott-Young, A. Thoracic Intercostal Nerve Blocks Reduce Opioid Consumption and Length of Stay in Patients Undergoing Implant-Based Breast Reconstruction. *Plast. Reconstr. Surg.* **2015**, *136*, 584e–591e. [CrossRef] [PubMed]
2. Lovich-Sapola, J.; Smith, C.E.; Brandt, C.P. Postoperative pain control. *Surg. Clin. N. Am.* **2015**, *95*, 301–318. [CrossRef] [PubMed]
3. Tasmuth, T.; Kataja, M.; Blomqvist, C.; von Smitten, K.; Kalso, E. Treatment-related factors predisposing to chronic pain in patients with breast cancer—A multivariate approach. *Acta Oncol.* **1997**, *36*, 625–630. [CrossRef]
4. Lanier, S.T.; Lewis, K.C.; Kendall, M.C.; Vieira, B.L.; De Oliveira, G., Jr.; Nader, A.; Kim, J.Y.S.; Alghoul, M. Intraoperative Nerve Blocks Fail to Improve Quality of Recovery after Tissue Expander Breast Reconstruction: A Prospective, Double-Blinded, Randomized, Placebo-Controlled Clinical Trial. *Plast. Reconstr. Surg.* **2018**, *141*, 590–597. [CrossRef]
5. Cuomo, R.; Zerini, I.; Botteri, G.; Barberi, L.; Nisi, G.; D'Aniello, C. Postsurgical pain related to breast implant: Reduction with lipofilling procedure. *In Vivo* **2014**, *28*, 993–996. [PubMed]
6. Cheville, A.L.; Tchou, J. Barriers to rehabilitation following surgery for primary breast cancer. *J. Surg. Oncol.* **2007**, *95*, 409–418. [CrossRef]
7. Vadivelu, N.; Schreck, M.; Lopez, J.; Kodumudi, G.; Narayan, D. Pain after mastectomy and breast reconstruction. *Am. Surg.* **2008**, *74*, 285–296.
8. De Oliveira, G.S., Jr.; Bialek, J.M.; Nicosia, L.; McCarthy, R.J.; Chang, R.; Fitzgerald, P.; Kim, J.Y. Lack of association between breast reconstructive surgery and the development of chronic pain after mastectomy: A propensity matched retrospective cohort analysis. *Breast* **2014**, *23*, 329–333. [CrossRef]
9. Mc, C.J. Anesthesia for radical mastectomy with intravenous pentothal sodium and intercostal nerve block. *N. Engl. J. Med.* **1946**, *235*, 295–298.
10. Kang, C.M.; Kim, W.J.; Yoon, S.H.; Cho, C.B.; Shim, J.S. Postoperative Pain Control by Intercostal Nerve Block After Augmentation Mammoplasty. *Aesthetic. Plast. Surg.* **2017**, *41*, 1031–1036. [CrossRef]
11. Vemula, R.; Kutzin, M.; Greco, G.; Kutzin, T. The use of intercostal nerve blocks for implant-based breast surgery. *Plast. Reconstr. Surg.* **2013**, *132*, 178e–180e. [CrossRef] [PubMed]
12. Kamali, P.; Koolen, P.G.; Ibrahim, A.M.; Paul, M.A.; Dikmans, R.E.; Schermerhorn, M.L.; Lee, B.T.; Lin, S.J. Analyzing Regional Differences over a 15-Year Trend of One-Stage versus Two-Stage Breast Reconstruction in 941,191 Postmastectomy Patients. *Plast. Reconstr. Surg.* **2016**, *138*, 1e–14e. [CrossRef] [PubMed]
13. Sisti, A.; Huayllani, M.T.; Boczar, D.; Restrepo, D.J.; Spaulding, A.C.; Emmanuel, G.; Bagaria, S.P.; McLaughlin, S.A.; Parker, A.S.; Forte, A.J. Breast cancer in women: A descriptive analysis of the national cancer database. *Acta Biomed.* **2020**, *91*, 332–341.
14. Cuomo, R. Submuscular and Pre-Pectoral ADM Assisted Immediate Breast Reconstruction: A Literature Review. *Medicina* **2020**, *56*, 256. [CrossRef]
15. Serrurier, L.C.; Rayne, S.; Venter, M.; Benn, C.A. Direct-to-Implant Breast Reconstruction without the Use of an Acellular Dermal Matrix Is Cost Effective and Oncologically Safe. *Plast. Reconstr. Surg.* **2017**, *139*, 809–817. [CrossRef]
16. Park, B.Y.; Hong, S.E.; Hong, M.K.; Woo, K.J. The influence of contralateral breast augmentation on the development of complications in direct-to-implant breast reconstruction. *J. Plast. Reconstr. Aesthet. Surg.* **2020**. [CrossRef]

17. Safran, T.; Al-Halabi, B.; Viezel-Mathieu, A.; Boileau, J.F.; Dionisopoulos, T. Direct-to-Implant, Prepectoral Breast Reconstruction: A Single-Surgeon Experience with 201 Consecutive Patients. *Plast. Reconstr. Surg.* **2020**, *145*, 686e–696e. [CrossRef]
18. Srinivasa, D.R.; Garvey, P.B.; Qi, J.; Hamill, J.B.; Kim, H.M.; Pusic, A.L.; Kronowitz, S.J.; Wilkins, E.G.; Butler, C.E.; Clemens, M.W. Direct-to-Implant versus Two-Stage Tissue Expander/Implant Reconstruction: 2-Year Risks and Patient-Reported Outcomes from a Prospective, Multicenter Study. *Plast. Reconstr. Surg.* **2017**, *140*, 869–877. [CrossRef]
19. Charlson, M.E.; Pompei, P.; Ales, K.L.; MacKenzie, C.R. A new method of classifying prognostic comorbidity in longitudinal studies: Development and validation. *J. Chronic. Dis.* **1987**, *40*, 373–383. [CrossRef]
20. Deyo, R.A.; Cherkin, D.C.; Ciol, M.A. Adapting a clinical comorbidity index for use with ICD-9-CM administrative databases. *J. Clin. Epidemiol.* **1992**, *45*, 613–619. [CrossRef]
21. Woo, K.J.; Kang, B.Y.; Min, J.J.; Park, J.W.; Kim, A.; Oh, K.S. Postoperative pain control by preventive intercostal nerve block under direct vision followed by catheter-based infusion of local analgesics in rib cartilage harvest for auricular reconstruction in children with microtia: A randomized controlled trial. *J. Plast. Reconstr. Aesthet. Surg.* **2016**, *69*, 1203–1210. [CrossRef]
22. Butz, D.R.; Shenaq, D.S.; Rundell, V.L.; Kepler, B.; Liederbach, E.; Thiel, J.; Pesce, C.; Murphy, G.S.; Sisco, M.; Howard, M.A. Postoperative Pain and Length of Stay Lowered by Use of Exparel in Immediate, Implant-Based Breast Reconstruction. *Plast. Reconstr. Surg. Glob. Open* **2015**, *3*, e391. [CrossRef]
23. Glenesk, N.L.; Lopez, P.P. Anatomy, Thorax, Intercostal Nerves. In *StatPearls*; StatPearls Publishing: Treasure Island, FL, USA, 2020.
24. Baxter, C.S.; Ajib, F.A.; Fitzgerald, B.M. Intercostal Nerve Block. In *StatPearls*; StatPearls Publishing: Treasure Island, FL, USA, 2020.
25. Hohmann, E.L.; Elde, R.P.; Rysavy, J.A.; Einzig, S.; Gebhard, R.L. Innervation of periosteum and bone by sympathetic vasoactive intestinal peptide-containing nerve fibers. *Science* **1986**, *232*, 868–871. [CrossRef] [PubMed]
26. Ellender, G.; Feik, S.A.; Carach, B.J. Periosteal structure and development in a rat caudal vertebra. *J. Anat.* **1988**, *158*, 173–187.
27. Mach, D.B.; Rogers, S.D.; Sabino, M.C.; Luger, N.M.; Schwei, M.J.; Pomonis, J.D.; Keyser, C.P.; Clohisy, D.R.; Adams, D.J.; O'Leary, P.; et al. Origins of skeletal pain: Sensory and sympathetic innervation of the mouse femur. *Neuroscience* **2002**, *113*, 155–166. [CrossRef]
28. Hwang, E.G.; Lee, Y. Effectiveness of intercostal nerve block for management of pain in rib fracture patients. *J. Exerc. Rehabil.* **2014**, *10*, 241–244. [CrossRef] [PubMed]
29. Chartier, S.R.; Thompson, M.L.; Longo, G.; Fealk, M.N.; Majuta, L.A.; Mantyh, P.W. Exuberant sprouting of sensory and sympathetic nerve fibers in nonhealed bone fractures and the generation and maintenance of chronic skeletal pain. *Pain* **2014**, *155*, 2323–2336. [CrossRef] [PubMed]
30. Maruccia, M.; Mazzocchi, M.; Dessy, L.A.; Onesti, M.G. One-stage breast reconstruction techniques in elderly patients to preserve quality of life. *Eur. Rev. Med. Pharm. Sci.* **2016**, *20*, 5058–5066.
31. Cattelani, L.; Polotto, S.; Arcuri, M.F.; Pedrazzi, G.; Linguadoca, C.; Bonati, E. One-Step Prepectoral Breast Reconstruction With Dermal Matrix-Covered Implant Compared to Submuscular Implantation: Functional and Cost Evaluation. *Clin. Breast Cancer* **2018**, *18*, e703–e711. [CrossRef] [PubMed]
32. Walia, G.S.; Aston, J.; Bello, R.; Mackert, G.A.; Pedreira, R.A.; Cho, B.H.; Carl, H.M.; Rada, E.M.; Rosson, G.D.; Sacks, J.M. Prepectoral Versus Subpectoral Tissue Expander Placement: A Clinical and Quality of Life Outcomes Study. *Plast. Reconstr. Surg. Glob. Open* **2018**, *6*, e1731. [CrossRef]
33. McCarthy, C.M.; Lee, C.N.; Halvorson, E.G.; Riedel, E.; Pusic, A.L.; Mehrara, B.J.; Disa, J.J. The use of acellular dermal matrices in two-stage expander/implant reconstruction: A multicenter, blinded, randomized controlled trial. *Plast. Reconstr. Surg.* **2012**, *130*, 57S–66S. [CrossRef] [PubMed]
34. Baker, B.G.; Irri, R.; MacCallum, V.; Chattopadhyay, R.; Murphy, J.; Harvey, J.R. A Prospective Comparison of Short-Term Outcomes of Subpectoral and Prepectoral Strattice-Based Immediate Breast Reconstruction. *Plast. Reconstr. Surg.* **2018**, *141*, 1077–1084. [CrossRef] [PubMed]
35. Moore, D.C. Intercostal nerve block for postoperative somatic pain following surgery of thorax and upper abdomen. *Br. J. Anaesth.* **1975**, *47*, 284–286. [PubMed]
36. Nunn, J.F.; Slavin, G. Posterior intercostal nerve block for pain relief after cholecystectomy. Anatomical basis and efficacy. *Br. J. Anaesth.* **1980**, *52*, 253–260. [CrossRef] [PubMed]

37. Mc, C.R.; Zollinger, R.; Lenahan, N.E. A clinical study of the effect of intercostal nerve block with nupercaine in oil following upper abdominal surgery. *Surg. Gynecol. Obstet.* **1948**, *86*, 680–686.
38. Schnabel, A.; Reichl, S.U.; Kranke, P.; Pogatzki-Zahn, E.M.; Zahn, P.K. Efficacy and safety of paravertebral blocks in breast surgery: A meta-analysis of randomized controlled trials. *Br. J. Anaesth.* **2010**, *105*, 842–852. [CrossRef]
39. Schwemmer, U. Breast surgery and peripheral blocks. Is it worth it? *Curr. Opin. Anaesthesiol.* **2020**, *33*, 311–315. [CrossRef]
40. Blanco, R.; Fajardo, M.; Parras Maldonado, T. Ultrasound description of Pecs II (modified Pecs I): A novel approach to breast surgery. *Rev. Esp. Anestesiol. Reanim.* **2012**, *59*, 470–475. [CrossRef]

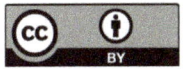

© 2020 by the authors. Licensee MDPI, Basel, Switzerland. This article is an open access article distributed under the terms and conditions of the Creative Commons Attribution (CC BY) license (http://creativecommons.org/licenses/by/4.0/).

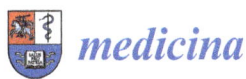

Article

Disparities in Access to Autologous Breast Reconstruction

David J. Restrepo [1], Maria T. Huayllani [1], Daniel Boczar [1], Andrea Sisti [2], Minh-Doan T. Nguyen [3], Jordan J. Cochuyt [4], Aaron C. Spaulding [4], Brian D. Rinker [1], Galen Perdikis [5] and Antonio J. Forte [1],*

1. Division of Plastic Surgery, Mayo Clinic, Jacksonville, FL 32224, USA; rpo20@hotmail.com (D.J.R.); maria.t.huayllanip@gmail.com (M.T.H.); danielboczar92@gmail.com (D.B.); rinker.brian@mayo.edu (B.D.R.)
2. Department of Plastic Surgery, Cleveland Clinic, OH 44195, USA; asisti6@gmail.com
3. Division of Plastic Surgery, Mayo Clinic, Rochester, MN 55905, USA; Nguyen.Minh-Doan@mayo.edu
4. Department of Health Science Research, Mayo Clinic, Jacksonville, FL 32224, USA; cochuyt.jordan@mayo.edu (J.J.C.); Spaulding.Aaron@mayo.edu (A.C.S.)
5. Department of Plastic Surgery, Vanderbilt University Medical Center, Nashville, TN 37232, USA; galen.perdikis@vanderbilt.edu
* Correspondence: forte.antonio@mayo.edu; Tel.: +1-9049532073

Received: 5 May 2020; Accepted: 4 June 2020; Published: 8 June 2020

Abstract: *Background and objectives:* This study aimed to determine if age, race, region, insurance, and comorbidities affect the type of breast reconstruction that patients receive. *Materials and methods:* This analysis used the Florida Inpatient Discharge Dataset from 1 January 2013 to 30 September 2017, which contains deidentified patient-level administrative data from all acute care hospitals in the state of Florida. We included female patients, diagnosed with breast cancer, who underwent mastectomy and a subsequent breast reconstruction. We performed an χ^2 test and logistic regression in this analysis. *Results:* On the multivariable analysis, we found that age, race, patient region, insurance payer, and Elixhauser score were all variables that significantly affected the type of reconstruction that patients received. Our results show that African American (odds ratio (OR): 0.68, 95% CI: 0.58–0.78, $p < 0.001$) and Hispanic or Latino (OR: 0.82, 95% CI: 0.72–0.93, $p = 0.003$) patients have significantly lower odds of receiving implant reconstruction when compared to white patients. Patients with Medicare (OR: 1.57, 95% CI: 1.33–1.86, $p < 0.001$) had significantly higher odds and patients with Medicaid (OR: 0.61, 95% CI: 0.51–0.74, $p < 0.001$) had significantly lower odds of getting autologous reconstruction when compared to patients with commercial insurance. *Conclusions:* Our study demonstrated that, in the state of Florida over the past years, variables, such as race, region, insurance, and comorbidities, play an important role in choosing the reconstruction modality. More efforts are needed to eradicate disparities and give all patients, despite their race, insurance payer, or region, equal access to health care.

Keywords: breast cancer; breast reconstruction; autologous reconstruction; disparities; public health; Florida

---

1. Introduction

The United States has 3.5 million breast cancer survivors [1]. With an estimated 279,100 new breast cancer diagnoses for 2020 and a steady decrease in mortality, the number of survivors is expected to increase [2,3].

Although lifesaving, mastectomy is a procedure that can cause significant psychological stress in patients who require it [4]. To improve this burden, breast reconstruction has become an important source of hope for these women. Women who receive breast reconstruction have shown improvement in health-related quality of life [4], while sexuality has been shown to be worse in patients who do not receive postmastectomy breast reconstruction [5].

As breast reconstruction rates increase [6], and with laws that make the procedure more widely available to the US population [7], new procedures have been developed and have proven to be as good, or better, than previous procedures. Breast reconstruction techniques currently available can be divided into autologous tissue-based or implant-based techniques [8]. Implant-based reconstruction is the most common type of reconstruction; however, women who receive autologous reconstruction have shown a higher rate of satisfaction [9].

The type of reconstruction used for a patient who received a mastectomy should be based on multiple factors; patient preference, age, weight, comorbidities, shape and size of the breast, mastectomy scar, surgeon experience, and cost should all be taken into account when selecting a reconstructive technique. However, factors, such as race, region, and insurance, should not be factors that affect the type of reconstruction. Equality is one of the main goals of the healthcare system, and disparities should not be present in any aspect of medicine. It has been reported that African American race is the most clinically significant predictor of autologous breast reconstruction and there is little data regarding the Hispanic population. With this study, we aimed to analyze the Florida Inpatient Discharge Dataset (FIDD) to see if factors, such as age, race, region, insurance, and comorbidities, have an effect on the type of breast reconstruction received by postmastectomy patients in Florida.

2. Materials and Methods

2.1. Data Source

This analysis used the FIDD, which contains deidentified patient-level administrative data from all acute care hospitals in the state of Florida.

2.2. Population and Variables

We included female patients who were 18 years or older, diagnosed with breast cancer, who underwent an elective reconstructive surgery involving either an implant or an autologous procedure from 1 January 2013 to 30 September 2017. We excluded male patients, and subjects who were enrolled on Medicaid but were less than 65 years old. The inclusion and exclusion of our population is further depicted in Figure 1.

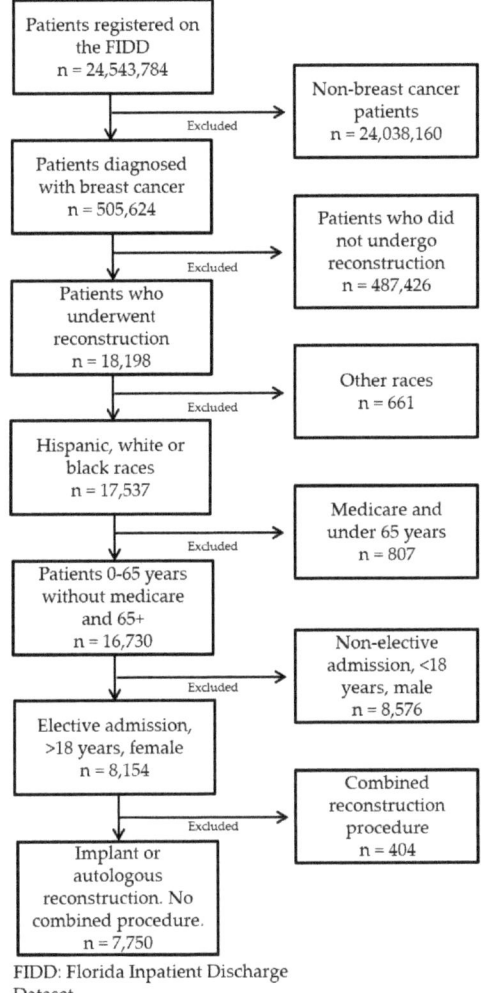

FIDD: Florida Inpatient Discharge Dataset

Figure 1. Inclusion and exclusion criteria.

2.3. Dependent Variables

The dependent variable for this analysis was whether the patient had an implant procedure or an autologous procedure (i.e., free, pedicled). The surgical procedures were defined by the International Classification of Diseases-9 (ICD) and ICD-10 codes.

2.4. Independent Variables

Patient characteristics, including age, race/ethnicity, region, insurance payer type, and comorbidities, were included as covariates. Race and ethnicity were categorized as white, black or African American, and Hispanic or Latino. Insurance payer type was categorized as Medicare (including Medicare Managed Care Patient), Medicaid (including Medicaid Managed Care Patient), commercial, or other (including self-pay or non-payment). Patients' regional locations were based on the seven regions of the Florida Department of Transportation, and indications of rurality were defined by the Florida Department of Health. We collapsed patient regions into North, South, and Central to allow for an acceptable amount of statistical power for the multivariable models. The Elixhauser score was used to indicate whether patients had comorbidities.

2.5. Analysis

Data were described as frequency and percentage or median and range. Pearson χ^2 and Kruskal–Wallis tests were used to compare categorical and continuous variables. The first statistical model focused on disparities among patients who received an implant or a flap procedure. We used multivariable logistic regression and summarized the data using odds ratios (ORs). Furthermore, 95% Confidence Intervals (CIs) were used to show the strength of the association between each of the different comparisons. All tests of significance were two-sided, and p values were reported. The level of statistical significance was set at α less than 0.05. Analyses were preformed using SAS, version 9.4 (SAS Institute Inc. Cary, NC, USA).

3. Results

A total of 7750 patients underwent postmastectomy breast reconstruction during the study period and met our inclusion criteria for the study. Table 1 outlines their demographic characteristics and Elixhauser Comorbidity Index score by type of reconstruction. Significant differences were found in all the groups. In our cohort, 4944 (68.7%) were white, 882 (12.3%) African American, and 1368 (19.0%) Hispanic or Latino. While most patients (7080 (95.1%)) had insurance, (361 (4.9%)) did not. There were a higher number of patients with no comorbidities (4185 (56.2%)) than patients with at least one comorbid condition (3256 (43.8%)), as calculated with the Elixhauser score.

Table 1. Surgical population's descriptive statistics for breast cancer patients.

Variable	Flap (n = 2809)	Implant (n = 4632)	Total (n = 7441)	p Value
Age	54.0 (20.0–93.0)	53.0 (21.0–87.0)	53.0 (20.0–93.0)	<0.0001 [1]
Year				<0.0001 [2]
2013	752 (26.8%)	1319 (28.5%)	2071 (27.8%)	
2014	765 (27.2%)	1147 (24.8%)	1912 (25.7%)	
2015	685 (24.4%)	1004 (21.7%)	1689 (22.7%)	
2016	382 (13.6%)	821 (17.7%)	1203 (16.2%)	
2017	225 (8.0%)	341 (7.4%)	566 (7.6%)	
Race				<0.0001 [2]
White	1798 (66.2%)	3146 (70.2%)	4944 (68.7%)	
Black or African American	400 (14.7%)	482 (10.8%)	882 (12.3%)	
Hispanic or Latino	517 (19.0%)	851 (19.0%)	1368 (19.0%)	
Patient Region				<0.0001 [2]
South Florida	1257 (46.1%)	2465 (54.3%)	3722 (51.2%)	
North Florida	605 (22.2%)	781 (17.2%)	1386 (19.1%)	
Central Florida	867 (31.8%)	1294 (28.5%)	2161 (29.7%)	
Patient Insurance Payer				<0.0001 [2]
Medicare	479 (17.1%)	839 (18.1%)	1318 (17.7%)	
Medicaid	238 (8.5%)	267 (5.8%)	505 (6.8%)	
Commercial	1916 (68.2%)	3341 (72.1%)	5257 (70.6%)	
Other	176 (6.3%)	185 (4.0%)	361 (4.9%)	
Elixhauser Score				<0.0001 [2]
No	1445 (51.4%)	2740 (59.2%)	4185 (56.2%)	
Yes	1364 (48.6%)	1892 (40.8%)	3256 (43.8%)	

Statistical tests of difference: [1] Kruskal–Wallis, [2] χ2. Statistics reported: Continuous variables were summarized with the median (range).

Using multivariable analysis, we found that age, race, patient region, insurance payer, and Elixhauser score were all variables that significantly affected the type of reconstruction that patients received (Table 2). The results show that both African American (OR: 0.68, 95% CI: 0.58–0.78, $p < 0.001$) and Hispanic or Latino (OR: 0.82, 95% CI: 0.72–0.93, $p = 0.003$) races have significantly lower odds of receiving implant reconstruction when compared to white patients. Interestingly, insurance showed mixed results; patients with Medicare (OR: 1.57, 95% CI: 1.33–1.86, $p < 0.001$) had significantly higher odds while patients with Medicaid (OR: 0.61, 95% CI: 0.51–0.74, $p < 0.001$) had significantly lower odds of getting implant reconstruction when compared to patients with commercial insurance. Patients with comorbidities, defined as an Elixhauser score greater than 0, were also found to have lower odds of implant reconstruction when compared to patients without comorbidities (OR: 0.80, 95% CI: 0.72–0.88, $p < 0.001$).

Table 2. Odds ratio of receiving implant breast reconstruction.

Variable	Implant vs. Flap (Ref)	
	OR (95% CI)	p Value
Age (10-year increase)	0.79 (0.75, 0.84)	<0.0001
Race	Overall Test of Difference: $p < 0.0001$	
White	1.00 (Ref)	N/A
Black or African American	0.67 (0.57, 0.78)	<0.0001
Hispanic or Latino	0.81 (0.71, 0.92)	
Patient Region	Overall Test of Difference: $p < 0.0001$	
North Florida	1.00 (Ref)	N/A
South Florida	1.61 (1.40, 1.83)	<0.0001
Central Florida	1.17 (1.02, 1.35)	
Patient Insurance Payer	Overall Test of Difference: $p < 0.0001$	
Commercial	1.00 (Ref)	N/A
Medicare	1.59 (1.34, 1.89)	<0.0001
Medicaid	0.62 (0.51, 0.75)	<0.0001
Other	0.64 (0.51, 0.80)	
Elixhauser Score		
No	1.00 (Ref)	N/A
Yes	0.75 (0.68, 0.82)	<0.0001

Abbreviations: N/A, not applicable; OR, odds ratio; Ref, reference.

Our multivariable analysis comparing the two types of autologous reconstruction (flap and pedicled flap) versus implant-based reconstruction alone also showed significant associations between the studied variables (Table 3). In terms of race, African Americans showed lower odds of getting implant reconstruction versus any type of flap when compared to white patients (implant versus free flap (OR: 0.61, 95% CI: 0.51, 0.74, $p < 0.001$) and versus pedicled flap (OR: 0.61, 95% CI: 0.44, 0.88, $p = 0.007$). On the contrary, there was no significant difference for Hispanic or Latino patients in implant versus pedicled flap reconstruction (OR: 0.96, 95% CI: 0.70, 1.31, $p = 0.79$) when compared to white patients.

Table 3. Logistic regression comparing different types of autologous vs. implant reconstruction.

Variable	Implant vs. Free Flap (Ref)		Implant vs. Pedicled Flap (Ref)	
	OR (95% CI)	p Value	OR (95% CI)	p Value
Age	0.81 (0.75, 0.88)	<0.0001	0.63 (0.54, 0.72)	<0.0001
Race	Overall Test of Difference: $p < 0.0001$		Overall Test of Difference: $p = 0.009$	
White	1.00 (Ref)	N/A	1.00 (Ref)	N/A
Black or African American	0.61 (0.51, 0.74)	<0.0001	0.61 (0.44, 0.84)	0.003
Hispanic or Latino	0.64 (0.55, 0.76)	<0.0001	0.97 (0.72, 1.31)	0.85
Patient Region	Overall Test of Difference: $p < 0.0001$		Overall Test of Difference: $p < 0.0001$	
North Florida	1.00 (Ref)	N/A	1.00 (Ref)	N/A
South Florida	2.09 (1.78, 2.45)	<0.0001	0.82 (0.58, 1.17)	0.27
Central Florida	2.11 (1.77, 2.52)	<0.0001	0.46 (0.32, 0.65)	<0.0001
Patient Insurance Payer	Overall Test of Difference: $p < 0.0001$		Overall Test of Difference: $p < 0.0001$	
Commercial	1.00 (Ref)	N/A	1.00 (Ref)	N/A
Medicare	2.71 (2.13, 3.44)	<0.0001	1.48 (1.03, 2.12)	0.035
Medicaid	0.93 (0.72, 1.21)	0.58	0.36 (0.25, 0.52)	<0.0001
Other	0.66 (0.51, 0.87)	0.003	0.66 (0.39, 1.10)	0.11
Elixhauser Score	Overall Test of Difference: $p < 0.0001$		Overall Test of Difference: $p = 0.0004$	
No	1.00 (Ref)	N/A	1.00 (Ref)	N/A
Yes	0.60 (0.53, 0.68)	<0.0001	1.75 (1.38, 2.22)	<0.0001

Abbreviations: N/A, not applicable; OR, odds ratio; Ref, reference.

4. Discussion

Breast cancer incidence is increasing [3]. Throughout their lifetime, breast cancer will affect one in every eight women in the United States [10]. Although breast conservation therapy remains an option, many of these women instead undergo mastectomy with or without breast reconstruction [11–15]. Efforts have been made nationally to make breast reconstruction more available to patients who undergo mastectomy. Evidence has shown an increase in the rate of breast reconstruction, which is a step forward in the physical and psychological treatment of breast cancer [16]. However, there are few studies of the disparities in access to autologous breast reconstruction in the United States [11,17–19], and none in Florida, where there is a larger Hispanic population than in most of states. The importance of this study is that it addresses this gap in the literature and will aid public health agencies to understand the factors that influence access to autologous breast reconstruction.

Despite not having a consensus on whether implant- or autologous-based reconstruction is better for patients, autologous-based reconstruction is currently recognized as the best option by providing the patient with a more natural look and feel [8]. When it comes to selecting the type of reconstruction a patient should receive, race, region, and insurance should not be determining factors.

Our results show that, even when corrected for confounders, some of these variables were significant when deciding what type of reconstruction patients received. Minorities, such as African American or Hispanic (Latino), had lower odds of receiving implant breast reconstruction, which implies that they received more autologous reconstruction. These results were expected, since despite lower rates of postmastectomy breast reconstruction in black patients when compared to white patients [17], it has already been shown that black patients have a higher rate of autologous breast reconstruction [11,17,18].

Sergesketter et al. [19] reported that black race (non-Hispanic) and Hispanic ethnicity had a lower likelihood of receiving breast reconstruction when compared to white patients. However, they also found that these two groups of patients were more likely to receive autologous than implant-based reconstruction.

Moreover, three studies found that black patients had a higher rate of autologous breast reconstruction when compared to their white counterparts [11,17,18]. One study found no significant difference between the groups [20].

Our results are in concordance with these studies and further contribute to the available literature on this subject. However, none of these studies identified the causality for these results. Unfortunately, disparities affecting breast cancer patients are not limited to autologous reconstruction. Our group has shown that the rate of breast reconstruction, refusal of surgical treatment, and the survival of male patients with breast cancer has also been shown to be affected by ethnic and demographic characteristics [21–24].

It was reported in two studies that postmastectomy breast reconstruction decreases the probability of depression and improves emotional, social, and physical functionality. Women who do not receive postmastectomy breast reconstruction have worse functionality on the mentioned aspects [5,25]. Although implant-based reconstruction is more common, a recent study published by Fracon and colleagues [9] showed that women who received autologous breast reconstruction showed a higher degree of satisfaction using the BREAST-Q module ($p = 0.00596$), psychosocial well-being module ($p = 0.04$), and sexual well-being module ($p = 0.00068$).

Despite having a longer operating time and more incisions, autologous breast reconstruction, such as the deep inferior epigastric (DIEP) flap, has been found to have fewer serious adverse effects leading to reconstruction failure or unpleasant aesthetic results when compared to tissue expander implant-based reconstruction [26].

Interestingly, Fischer and colleagues [27] conducted a study in which adverse effects were compared in patients receiving free flap reconstruction versus tissue expander and implant reconstruction in a high-volume institution. On an average two-year follow-up, a 98.8% success rate was reported with free flap reconstruction, while a 94.4% success rate was reported with tissue expander reconstruction. Interestingly, the free flap was also associated with a lower rate of unplanned reoperation (5.8% vs. 16.8%; $p = 0.002$) [27]. These results are in line with Spear and colleagues' results [28]. In contrast, Mioton and colleagues [29], using the National Surgical Quality Improvement Project Dataset, reported higher rates of failure in autologous reconstruction (3.13% vs. 0.85%; $p < 0.001$); however, it is important to note that the follow-up period included only 30 days, showing that during the first 30 days, autologous reconstruction can present a higher rate of failure. Autologous reconstruction is also known to be a more complicated procedure, requiring a longer operating time. Due to the higher complexity of autologous breast reconstruction, its costs are higher. However, Fischer and colleagues [27] reported that even though autologous reconstruction has a higher upfront operation cost, it is more cost efficient over time. Other studies have supported this result, especially over time [30,31].

Surgeon reimbursement can be a matter of discussion, too, as it is sometimes believed that autologous reconstruction is not cost effective for practitioners. Sando and colleagues [32] reported that contrary to the perceptions, the complex reconstructive procedures that patients undergo for autologous reconstruction consistently generated more revenue and an hourly reimbursement that showed no statistical difference ($1053 vs. $947; $p = 0.72$). Other studies have demonstrated that autologous reconstruction is also more cost-efficient and profitable for hospitals [29,33].

Despite all this information, implant reconstruction is more common than autologous reconstruction. National trends show an increase in implant-based breast reconstruction and a decrease in autologous reconstruction [34]. However, plastic surgeons who practice at academic university programs do not follow the same trends [34]. Implant-based reconstruction rates, which have typically trended up, now show a plateau in academic hospitals, while the rate of autologous reconstruction, more specifically the DIEP flap, has increased [34].

Considering the previously mentioned information in favor of autologous breast reconstruction, it is interesting to see that in Florida, black and Hispanic patients receive a lower proportion of implant reconstructions, suggesting a higher rate of autologous reconstruction. It was also shown that patients with Medicaid who receive reconstruction have lower odds of getting implant reconstruction, implying a higher proportion of autologous reconstruction when compared to commercial insurance. On the contrary, patients with Medicare had lower odds of receiving autologous breast reconstruction, showing that there are disparities, even among the two government insurance types.

This study has several limitations. Our analysis was done using the FIDD because it captures 100% of the patients with breast cancer treated in Florida health institutions. Due to the nature of databases, the fidelity of the information can be affected by incorrect or incomplete reports. Furthermore, the FIDD registers every event separately, meaning that if the same patient has two outpatient visits or two different reconstruction procedures, her cases would be registered as two separate cases. Additionally, a large proportion of the patients in the database were excluded due to our inclusion and exclusion criteria; however, the number of studied patients was substantial and allowed for multivariable analyses.

5. Conclusions

Our study demonstrated that, in the state of Florida, variables, such as race, region, insurance, and comorbidities, seem to play an important role in selecting the reconstruction modality. More efforts are needed to eradicate disparities and give all patients, despite their race, insurance, or region, equal access to health care.

Author Contributions: Conceptualization, D.B.; Data curation, M.T.H. and J.J.C.; Formal analysis, A.C.S.; Funding acquisition, M.T.H.; Investigation, D.J.R. and A.S.; Methodology, D.J.R., A.S., J.J.C., A.C.S. and G.P.; Project administration, D.B.; Software, J.J.C. and A.C.S.; Supervision, M.-D.T.N., B.D.R., G.P. and A.J.F.; Writing—original draft, D.J.R.; Writing—review and editing, M.T.H., A.S., M.-D.T.N., B.D.R., G.P. and A.J.F. All authors have read and agreed to the published version of the manuscript.

Funding: This study was supported in part by the Center for Individualized Medicine and the Plastic Surgery Foundation.

Conflicts of Interest: All authors report no conflict of interests in this study.

References

1. Miller, K.D.; Siegel, R.L.; Lin, C.C.; Mariotto, A.B.; Kramer, J.L.; Rowland, J.H.; Stein, K.D.; Alteri, R.; Jemal, A. Cancer treatment and survivorship statistics, 2016. *CA Cancer J. Clin.* **2016**, *66*, 271–289. [CrossRef] [PubMed]
2. Siegel, R.L.; Miller, K.D.; Jemal, A. Cancer statistics, 2020. *CA Cancer J. Clin.* **2020**, *70*, 7–30. [CrossRef] [PubMed]
3. Sisti, A.; Huayllani, M.T.; Boczar, D.; Restrepo, D.J.; Spaulding, A.C.; Emmanuel, G.; Bagaria, S.P.; McLaughlin, S.A.; Parker, A.S.; Forte, A.J. Breast cancer in women: A descriptive analysis of the national cancer database. *Acta Biomed.* **2020**, *91*, 332–341. [PubMed]
4. Fanakidou, I.; Zyga, S.; Alikari, V.; Tsironi, M.; Stathoulis, J.; Theofilou, P. Mental health, loneliness, and illness perception outcomes in quality of life among young breast cancer patients after mastectomy: The role of breast reconstruction. *Qual. Life Res.* **2018**, *27*, 539–543. [CrossRef] [PubMed]
5. Trejo-Ochoa, J.L.; Maffuz-Aziz, A.; Said-Lemus, F.M.; Dominguez-Reyes, C.A.; Hernandez-Hernandez, B.; Villegas-Carlos, F.; Rodriguez-Cuevas, S. Impact on quality of life with breast reconstructive surgery after mastectomy for breast cancer. [Article in Spanish]. *Ginecol. Obstet. Mex.* **2013**, *81*, 510–518.
6. Panchal, H.; Matros, E. Current Trends in Postmastectomy Breast Reconstruction. *Plast. Reconstr. Surg.* **2017**, *140*, 7S–13S. [CrossRef]
7. Yang, R.L.; Newman, A.S.; Reinke, C.E.; Lin, I.C.; Karakousis, G.C.; Czerniecki, B.J.; Wu, L.C.; Kelz, R.R. Racial disparities in immediate breast reconstruction after mastectomy: Impact of state and federal health policy changes. *Ann. Surg. Oncol.* **2013**, *20*, 399–406. [CrossRef]
8. Leuzzi, S.; Stivala, A.; Shaff, J.B.; Maroccia, A.; Rausky, J.; Revol, M.; Bertrand, B.; Cristofari, S. Latissimus dorsi breast reconstruction with or without implants: A comparison between outcome and patient satisfaction. *J. Plast. Reconstr. Aesthet. Surg.* **2019**, *72*, 381–393. [CrossRef]
9. Fracon, S.; Renzi, N.; Manara, M.; Ramella, V.; Papa, G.; Arnez, Z.M. Patient Satisfaction After Breast Reconstruction: Implants vs. Autologous Tissues. *Acta Chir. Plast.* **2018**, *59*, 120–128.
10. DeSantis, C.; Ma, J.; Bryan, L.; Jemal, A. Breast cancer statistics, 2013. *CA Cancer J. Clin.* **2014**, *64*, 52–62. [CrossRef]
11. Alderman, A.K.; McMahon, L., Jr.; Wilkins, E.G. The national utilization of immediate and early delayed breast reconstruction and the effect of sociodemographic factors. *Plast. Reconstr. Surg.* **2003**, *111*, 695–703, discussion 704–705. [CrossRef]

12. Xie, Y.; Tang, Y.; Wehby, G.L. Federal Health Coverage Mandates and Health Care Utilization: The Case of the Women's Health and Cancer Rights Act and Use of Breast Reconstruction Surgery. *J. Womens Health (Larchmt)* **2015**, *24*, 655–662. [CrossRef]
13. Cordeiro, P.G. Breast reconstruction after surgery for breast cancer. *N. Engl. J. Med.* **2008**, *359*, 1590–1601. [CrossRef] [PubMed]
14. Wilkins, E.G.; Alderman, A.K. Breast reconstruction practices in north america: Current trends and future priorities. *Semin. Plast. Surg.* **2004**, *18*, 149–155. [CrossRef] [PubMed]
15. Guyomard, V.; Leinster, S.; Wilkinson, M. Systematic review of studies of patients' satisfaction with breast reconstruction after mastectomy. *Breast* **2007**, *16*, 547–567. [CrossRef]
16. Ilonzo, N.; Tsang, A.; Tsantes, S.; Estabrook, A.; Thu Ma, A.M. Breast reconstruction after mastectomy: A ten-year analysis of trends and immediate postoperative outcomes. *Breast* **2017**, *32*, 7–12. [CrossRef]
17. Offodile, A.C., 2nd; Tsai, T.C.; Wenger, J.B.; Guo, L. Racial disparities in the type of postmastectomy reconstruction chosen. *J. Surg. Res.* **2015**, *195*, 368–376. [CrossRef] [PubMed]
18. Albornoz, C.R.; Bach, P.B.; Pusic, A.L.; McCarthy, C.M.; Mehrara, B.J.; Disa, J.J.; Cordeiro, P.G.; Matros, E. The influence of sociodemographic factors and hospital characteristics on the method of breast reconstruction, including microsurgery: A U.S. population-based study. *Plast. Reconstr. Surg.* **2012**, *129*, 1071–1079. [CrossRef]
19. Sergesketter, A.R.; Thomas, S.M.; Lane, W.O.; Orr, J.P.; Shammas, R.L.; Fayanju, O.M.; Greenup, R.A.; Hollenbeck, S.T. Decline in Racial Disparities in Postmastectomy Breast Reconstruction: A Surveillance, Epidemiology, and End Results Analysis from 1998 to 2014. *Plast. Reconstr. Surg.* **2019**, *143*, 1560–1570. [CrossRef]
20. Rodby, K.A.; Danielson, K.K.; Shay, E.; Robinson, E.; Benjamin, M.; Antony, A.K. Trends in Breast Reconstruction by Ethnicity: An Institutional Review Centered on the Treatment of an Urban Population. *Am. Surg.* **2016**, *82*, 497–504.
21. Restrepo, D.J.; Boczar, D.; Huayllani, M.T.; Sisti, A.; Gabriel, E.; McLaughlin, S.A.; Bagaria, S.; Spaulding, A.C.; Rinker, B.D.; Forte, A.J. Influence of Race, Income, Insurance, and Education on the Rate of Breast Reconstruction. *Anticancer Res.* **2019**, *39*, 2969–2973. [CrossRef] [PubMed]
22. Restrepo, D.J.; Sisti, A.; Boczar, D.; Huayllani, M.T.; Fishe, J.; Gabriel, E.; McLaughlin, S.A.; Bagaria, S.; Spaulding, A.; Rinker, B.D.; et al. Characteristics of Breast Cancer Patients Who Refuse Surgery. *Anticancer Res.* **2019**, *39*, 4941–4945. [CrossRef] [PubMed]
23. Restrepo, D.J.; Boczar, D.; Huayllani, M.T.; Sisti, A.; McLaughlin, S.A.; Spaulding, A.; Parker, A.S.; Carter, R.E.; Leppin, A.L.; Forte, A.J. Survival Disparities in Male Patients With Breast Cancer. *Anticancer Res.* **2019**, *39*, 5669–5674. [CrossRef] [PubMed]
24. Boczar, D.; Restrepo, D.J.; Sisti, A.; Huayllani, M.T.; Spaulding, A.C.; Gabriel, E.; Bagaria, S.; McLaughlin, S.; Parker, A.S.; Forte, A.J. Influence of Facility Characteristics on Access to Breast Reconstruction: A 12-Year National Cancer Database Analysis. *Anticancer Res.* **2019**, *39*, 6881–6885. [CrossRef]
25. Ahn, S.H.; Park, B.W.; Noh, D.Y.; Nam, S.J.; Lee, E.S.; Lee, M.K.; Kim, S.H.; Lee, K.M.; Park, S.M.; Yun, Y.H. Health-related quality of life in disease-free survivors of breast cancer with the general population. *Ann. Oncol.* **2007**, *18*, 173–182. [CrossRef]
26. Lagares-Borrego, A.; Gacto-Sanchez, P.; Infante-Cossio, P.; Barrera-Pulido, F.; Sicilia-Castro, D.; Gomez-Cia, T. A comparison of long-term cost and clinical outcomes between the two-stage sequence expander/prosthesis and autologous deep inferior epigastric flap methods for breast reconstruction in a public hospital. *J. Plast. Reconstr. Aesthet. Surg.* **2016**, *69*, 196–205. [CrossRef]
27. Fischer, J.P.; Wes, A.M.; Nelson, J.A.; Basta, M.; Rohrbach, J.I.; Wu, L.C.; Serletti, J.M.; Kovach, S.J. Propensity-matched, longitudinal outcomes analysis of complications and cost: Comparing abdominal free flaps and implant-based breast reconstruction. *J. Am. Coll. Surg.* **2014**, *219*, 303–312. [CrossRef]
28. Spear, S.L.; Newman, M.K.; Bedford, M.S.; Schwartz, K.A.; Cohen, M.; Schwartz, J.S. A retrospective analysis of outcomes using three common methods for immediate breast reconstruction. *Plast. Reconstr. Surg.* **2008**, *122*, 340–347. [CrossRef]
29. Mioton, L.M.; Smetona, J.T.; Hanwright, P.J.; Seth, A.K.; Wang, E.; Bilimoria, K.Y.; Gaido, J.; Fine, N.A.; Kim, J.Y. Comparing thirty-day outcomes in prosthetic and autologous breast reconstruction: A multivariate analysis of 13.082 patients? *J. Plast. Reconstr. Aesthet. Surg.* **2013**, *66*, 917–925. [CrossRef]

30. Lista, F.; Ahmad, J. Evidence-based medicine: Augmentation mammaplasty. *Plast. Reconstr. Surg.* **2013**, *132*, 1684–1696. [CrossRef]
31. Bank, J.; Phillips, N.A.; Park, J.E.; Song, D.H. Economic analysis and review of the literature on implant-based breast reconstruction with and without the use of the acellular dermal matrix. *Aesth. Plast. Surg.* **2013**, *37*, 1194–1201. [CrossRef] [PubMed]
32. Sando, I.C.; Momoh, A.O.; Chung, K.C.; Kozlow, J.H. The Early Years of Practice: An Assessment of Operative Efficiency and Cost of Free Flap and Implant Breast Reconstruction at an Academic Institution. *J. Reconstr. Microsurg.* **2016**, *32*, 445–454. [CrossRef] [PubMed]
33. Hanwright, P.J.; Davila, A.A.; Hirsch, E.M.; Khan, S.A.; Fine, N.A.; Bilimoria, K.Y.; Kim, J.Y. The differential effect of BMI on prosthetic versus autogenous breast reconstruction: A multivariate analysis of 12.986 patients. *Breast* **2013**, *22*, 938–945. [CrossRef] [PubMed]
34. Dasari, C.R.; Gunther, S.; Wisner, D.H.; Cooke, D.T.; Gold, C.K.; Wong, M.S. Rise in microsurgical free-flap breast reconstruction in academic medical practices. *Ann. Plast. Surg.* **2015**, *74*, S62–S65. [CrossRef]

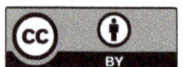

© 2020 by the authors. Licensee MDPI, Basel, Switzerland. This article is an open access article distributed under the terms and conditions of the Creative Commons Attribution (CC BY) license (http://creativecommons.org/licenses/by/4.0/).

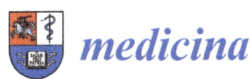

Review

Nipple–Areola Complex Reconstruction

Andrea Sisti

Department of Plastic Surgery, Cleveland Clinic, Cleveland, OH 44195, USA; asisti6@gmail.com

Received: 20 April 2020; Accepted: 10 June 2020; Published: 16 June 2020

Abstract: The reconstruction of the nipple–areola complex is the last step in the breast reconstruction process. Several techniques have been described over the years. The aim of this review is to provide clarity on the currently available reconstructive options.

Keywords: nipple reconstruction; areola reconstruction; breast reconstruction; nipple–areola reconstruction; local flap; skin graft

1. Introduction

Whenever possible, the surgeon spares the nipple areola complex (NAC) during breast demolition, through skin-sparing mastectomy or through nipple-sparing mastectomy [1]. In general, a tumor to nipple distance measured preoperatively by a digital mammogram of 2.5 cm or more is safe for NAC preservation in patients considered for breast conservation therapy [2].

When this is not possible, the areola–nipple complex is surgically removed together with the cancerous breast tissue and the nipple–areola complex is reconstructed afterward or in the same surgical session [3].

The reconstruction of the nipple–areola complex represents the final step of the breast reconstruction journey and it is generally performed four to six months after breast reconstruction [4–8]. The nipple–areola complex represents a very important anatomical part for the woman and the reconstruction has considerable aesthetic and psychological consequences [9–11].

Nevertheless, some women decline the reconstruction of the NAC after breast reconstruction [12]. Patients with later-stage cancer and a history of implant removal are less likely to have NAC reconstruction [12]. Satisfaction determinants are projection, color match, shape, size, texture, and position [13].

Several techniques have been proposed for the reconstruction [4–7,14–18]. Some authors have attempted to clarify the available surgical techniques for nipple–areola complex reconstruction. The first was Farhadi et al. [15] (Switzerland) in 2006, followed by Boccola et al. [14] (Australia) in 2010, Nimboriboonporn and Chuthapisith [17] (Thailand) in 2014 and Sisti et al. [5] (Italy) in 2016. In particular, Nimboriboonporn and Chuthapisith [17] proposed a first classification of nipple–areola reconstruction, according to the performed technique and to the type of material eventually grafted inside the neo-nipple. More recently (2018), Gougoutas et al. [16] published a quite comprehensive review on nipple–areola complex reconstruction.

It is important to distinguish between techniques used to reconstruct the nipple and techniques used to reconstruct the areola. Even though the nipple–areola is a complex, different techniques are performed to reconstruct the nipple and the areola. The literature on this topic is vast, but I will try my best to make it clear in this review.

2. Location of the Nipple and Areola Size

The location of the nipple on the reconstructed breast is a debated topic [19–21]. Pennisi et al. [20,21] proposed to place the new nipple 1/2 inch lateral to the mid-clavicular line on the sixth rib or interspace, while dr. Barnett [19] suggested to leave the decision about the new nipple–areola complex placement up to the patient.

Regarding the areola size, the choice is usually left to the patient if both the areolas have to be reconstructed, or the contralateral areola size is used as a model if only one areola needs to be reconstructed.

Laschuk et al. [22] recently proposed that the breast base width can be used to determine the ideal areolar size, using the areola: base width ratio of 0.29.

3. Nipple Reconstruction with Local Flap

The local flap is the most used technique for the reconstruction of the nipple [5,8,14–17]. This is a skin flap that usually includes the local skin and the superficial layer of the underlying subcutaneous tissue.

In 1946, Berson [23] firstly described the use of a local skin flap for nipple reconstruction. Each surgeon uses the flap technique that is most familiar with, since the superiority of one technique over the others has not been demonstrated [5,24].

The most commonly used flaps are the arrow flap [25,26], the C-V flap [27] and the C-H flap [3].

Some techniques involve the projecting of the central area of the areola with purse string sutures, overgrafts, and buried grafts [28]. New design flaps are continuously described [29,30].

The main issue is maintaining the nipple's projection [31] over time, since the new local flap tends to flatten. Sometimes the repetition of the same flap is necessary after the first surgery [32].

4. Use of Autologous/Allogenic/Synthetic Grafts to Improve Nipple Projection

To overcome the loss of projection, several material grafts have been proposed inside the new nipple: autologous tissue (fat [33], cartilage [25,34–38], derma [39]), allogeneic tissue (acellular dermal matrix [40,41], lyophilized allogeneic costal cartilage [42]), and synthetic materials (fillers [43–45] et al. [46,47]) can be grafted inside the nipple. Winocour et al. [18] have published an interesting review on this topic, concluding that the autologous tissue grafted inside the nipple has led to the best results.

More recently, Oliver et al. [46] focused their attention on allogeneic and alloplastic augmentation grafts in nipple–areola complex reconstruction in a systematic review, finding that the use of Ceratite (artificial bone) led to the highest complication rates [46].

Jankau et al. [48] proposed the use of a silicone rod inside the neo-nipple to enhance the projection over time, but the complications' rate was high (10/30 patients developed flap necrosis followed by rod removal).

Tierney et al. [49] and Collins et al. [50] described the use of the Biodesign Nipple Reconstruction Cylinder (a rolled cylinder of extracellular matrix collagen derived from porcine small intestinal submucosa) inside the nipple reconstructed using skin flaps, with positive outcomes.

A tightly rolled dermal graft [51] might also be used for nipple reconstruction as well, in order to improve the long-term maintenance of nipple projection.

5. Areola Reconstruction Using Skin Graft

The reconstruction of the areola can be performed with a skin graft from hyper-chromic skin areas, like the inguinal (the inner thigh skin), the axillary region or the labia minora skin [52].

In 1949, Adams [53] described the first areola reconstruction using a full-thickness skin graft (FTSG) from the labium minora. This surgical operation is easy to perform and the healing process in both the donor and recipient sites is generally fast. The complication rate associated with the use of the skin graft for the areola reconstruction is low but higher when compared to the tattoo [5].

The main issue associated with the use of a FTSG for the areola reconstruction is the fading of the pigmentation over time. It is not uncommon to perform the skin graft again, one to two years after the initial graft.

6. Nipple Sharing Technique for Nipple Reconstruction

This technique can be performed only in case of unilateral breast reconstruction. It is a skin graft from the contralateral nipple [54]. The surgical procedure is well described in a video recently published by Gougoutas et al. [16]. The nipple is divided in half on a sagittal plane and then the harvested half nipple is grafted on a previously de-epithelized circular skin area on the opposite breast [16].

The breastfeeding functionality can be preserved using a nipple-sharing technique that does not damage the anatomic structure of the donor nipple for breastfeeding [55]. This technique was described by Sakai and Taneda and consists of harvesting tissue by the circumcision method of nipple reduction and grafting the tissue in a spiral configuration [55].

The surgeon can choose to use no sutures after graft removal and letting the donor nipple heal spontaneously, minimizing scarring preserving the natural appearance and good sensitivity of the donor nipple [56].

7. Tattooing of the Nipple–Areola Complex

The tattoo of the nipple–areola complex is commonly performed four to six months after the surgical reconstruction of the nipple [5]. Nevertheless, the use of local flaps for nipple reconstruction and medical tattooing of the NAC in one session has been described [57].

The procedure is easy to perform in an outpatient setting and can be performed by a non-medical professional as well. It is a safe procedure [5] and leads to a high level of satisfaction [58,59]. Sometimes, just the areola is tattooed, for instance the nipple can be reconstructed using the nipple–sharing technique and the areola can be tattooed [60].

The tattoo can be made before the nipple reconstruction, but this may modify the final circular border of the areola after nipple reconstruction. However, the sequence of nipple reconstruction and tattooing has no significant effect on the projection of the reconstructed nipple [61].

Sasaki et al. [62] proposed four tips for tattooing procedures in nipple–areola complex reconstruction: blurring the areola margin, creating the illusion of the Montgomery glands (areolar bumps), adjusting the areola position to achieve symmetry and creating the illusion of the height of the nipple by using shading.

Some authors have proposed to have the tattoo done before surgery [5]. Furthermore, the reconstruction of the whole areola–nipple complex by 3-D tattoo is more and more widespread [59,63,64].

Post-tattooing complications are rare. Joseph et al. [65] recently reported a delayed hypersensitivity reaction around tattooed nipple areolar complexes in a 33-year-old female nonsmoker patient. Starnoni et al. [66] described a rare case of nipple–areolar complex partial necrosis following micropigmentation.

As for the FTSG, because of fading of the pigment, further tattooing may be required, and areolar color mismatch is another possible eventuality [52]. Allergic contact dermatitis of the breast secondary to pigment reaction related to the areola tattoo has also been described [67].

8. Other Techniques

External nipple–areola prosthetics made of silicone or other materials are another possible option for the reconstruction [68–72]. The use of internal nipple prosthesis [73] has been described as well, but is less common.

Dermoabrasion to re-create a nipple areola complex has been proposed by Cohen [74] in a black patient, resulting in a hyperpigmented area without the need for a skin graft. Furthermore, De Cholnoky [75] proposed the eversion of the navel to re-create the nipple when abdominal skin tissue is used to reconstruct the breast.

9. Projection

The loss of projection over time is the main issue after nipple reconstruction, even though the patient satisfaction and projection are not necessarily related, as observed by Jones and Erdmann [38].

Few et al. [31] observed a consistent 60% loss of intraoperative nipple projection in a study on 93 patients, with two years of follow-up. Lee et al. [61] found a mean loss of projection of 52.5–55.1% after six months.

In general, is advisable to build in the first place a nipple taller/bigger than the contralateral, since about 50% of projection is expected [5,17,61]. The local skin flap's thickness influences the neo-nipple projection, as observed by Ishii et al. [76].

The sequence of nipple reconstruction and tattooing does not affect the projection of the reconstructed nipple, as observed by Lee et al. [61] in a study on 394 reconstructed nipples. The use of graft augmentation showed a minor loss of nipple projection but might expose to an increased risk of complications [48].

10. Complications

In general, the incidence of complications is very low (0–11%) and the results in terms of patient satisfaction are remarkable [5,13,16,77].

The possible complications are nipple necrosis, tip loss, wound infection and wound breakdown [77]. Nipple necrosis is a rare event, due to the dual nature of the local flap. The local flap for nipple reconstruction is, in fact, a random skin flap that benefits also of imbibition from the underneath and surrounding skin areas (like skin grafts), given the very thin thickness of the skin flap itself. In the case of previous postmastectomy radiation, the reconstruction of the nipple is associated with an increased complication risk [77,78]. Implant-based breast reconstruction might be associated with higher rate of nipple reconstruction issues [77].

The local flap is the safest described technique for the nipple reconstruction [5]. The tattooing of the areola showed a lower number of complications compared to the areola reconstruction using a skin graft [5].

Fading after tattoo or after skin graft is common over time, therefore it is advisable to use a darker pigment for the tattoo or to choose a darker skin area as a place where to harvest the skin graft in the first place.

11. Conclusions

Nipple–areola complex reconstruction is a very important step in the breast reconstruction journey. A comprehensive understanding of the available options for reconstruction is of paramount importance for the plastic surgeon.

Funding: This research received no external funding.

Conflicts of Interest: The authors declare no conflict of interest.

References

1. Galimberti, V.; Vicini, E.; Corso, G.; Morigi, C.; Fontana, S.; Sacchini, V.; Veronesi, P. Nipple-sparing and skin-sparing mastectomy: Review of aims, oncological safety and contraindications. *Breast* **2017**, *34* (Suppl. 1), S82–S84. [CrossRef] [PubMed]
2. Augustine, P.; Ramesh, S.A.; Nair, R.K.; Sukumaran, R.; Jose, R.; Cherian, K.; Muralee, M.; Ahamad, I. Nipple Areola Complex Involvement in Invasive Carcinoma Breast. *Indian J. Surg. Oncol.* **2018**, *9*, 343–348. [CrossRef] [PubMed]
3. Yoon, J.S.; Chang, J.W.; Ahn, H.C.; Chung, M.S. Modified C-H flap for simultaneous nipple reconstruction during autologous breast reconstruction: Surgical tips for safety and cosmesis. *Medicine* **2018**, *97*, e12460. [CrossRef] [PubMed]
4. Cuomo, R.; Sisti, A.; Grimaldi, L.; D'Aniello, C. Modified Arrow Flap Technique for Nipple Reconstruction. *Breast J.* **2016**, *22*, 710–711. [CrossRef]
5. Sisti, A.; Grimaldi, L.; Tassinari, J.; Cuomo, R.; Fortezza, L.; Bocchiotti, M.A.; Roviello, F.; D'Aniello, C.; Nisi, G. Nipple-areola complex reconstruction techniques: A literature review. *Eur. J. Surg. Oncol. (EJSO)* **2016**, *42*, 441–465. [CrossRef]
6. Sisti, A.; Alfieri, E.P.; Brandi, C.; Nisi, G.; Grimaldi, L. Nipple-Areola Complex Reconstruction. *Plast. Reconstr. Surg.* **2018**, *142*, 793e. [CrossRef]
7. Sisti, A.; Tassinari, J.; Nisi, G.; Grimaldi, L. Autologous, Allogeneic, and Synthetic Augmentation Grafts in Nipple Reconstruction. *Plast. Reconstr. Surg.* **2016**, *138*, 936e–937e. [CrossRef]
8. Sisti, A.; Tassinari, J.; Cuomo, R.; Brandi, C.; Nisi, G.; Grimaldi, L.; D'Aniello, C. Nipple-Areola Complex Reconstruction. In *Nipple-Areolar Complex Reconstruction Principles and Clinical Techniques*; Shiffman, M.A., Ed.; Springer Science Publishing: Berlin/Heidelberg, Germany, 2017; pp. 359–368.
9. Goh, S.; Martin, N.; Pandya, A.; Cutress, R. Patient satisfaction following nipple-areolar complex reconstruction and tattooing. *J. Plast. Reconstr. Aesthetic Surg.* **2011**, *64*, 360–363. [CrossRef]
10. O Momoh, A.; Colakoglu, S.; De Blacam, C.; Yueh, J.H.; Lin, S.J.; Tobias, A.M.; Lee, B.T. The Impact of Nipple Reconstruction on Patient Satisfaction in Breast Reconstruction. *Ann. Plast. Surg.* **2012**, *69*, 389–393. [CrossRef]
11. Wellisch, D.K.; Schain, W.S.; Noone, R.B.; Little, J.W. The Psychological Contribution of Nipple Addition in Breast Reconstruction. *Plast. Reconstr. Surg.* **1987**, *80*, 699–704. [CrossRef]
12. Weissler, E.H.; Schnur, J.B.; Lamelas, A.M.; Cornejo, M.; Horesh, E.; Taub, P.J. The Necessity of the Nipple: Redefining Completeness in Breast Reconstruction. *Ann. Plast. Surg.* **2017**, *78*, 646–650. [CrossRef] [PubMed]
13. Jabor, M.A.; Shayani, P.; Collins, D.R.; Karas, T.; Cohen, B.E. Nipple-Areola Reconstruction: Satisfaction and Clinical Determinants. *Plast. Reconstr. Surg.* **2002**, *110*, 457–463. [CrossRef] [PubMed]
14. Boccola, M.; Savage, J.; Rozen, W.M.; Ashton, M.; Milner, C.; Rahdon, R.; Whitaker, I.S. Surgical Correction and Reconstruction of the Nipple-Areola Complex: Current Review of Techniques. *J. Reconstr. Microsurg.* **2010**, *26*, 589–600. [CrossRef]
15. Farhadi, J.; Maksvytyte, G.K.; Schaefer, D.J.; Pierer, G.; Scheufler, O. Reconstruction of the nipple-areola complex: An update. *J. Plast. Reconstr. Aesthetic Surg.* **2006**, *59*, 40–53. [CrossRef]
16. Gougoutas, A.J.; Said, H.K.; Um, G.; Chapin, A.; Mathes, D. Nipple-Areola Complex Reconstruction. *Plast. Reconstr. Surg.* **2018**, *141*, 404e–416e. [CrossRef]
17. Nimboriboonporn, A.; Chuthapisith, S. Nipple-areola complex reconstruction. *Gland. Surg.* **2014**, *3*, 35–42. [PubMed]
18. Winocour, S.; Saksena, A.; Oh, C.; Wu, P.S.; Laungani, A.; Baltzer, H.; Saint-Cyr, M. A Systematic Review of Comparison of Autologous, Allogeneic, and Synthetic Augmentation Grafts in Nipple Reconstruction. *Plast. Reconstr. Surg.* **2016**, *137*, 14e–23e. [CrossRef]
19. Barnett, A. Nipple-areola location in breast reconstruction: A simplified approach. *Plast. Reconstr. Surg.* **1990**, *85*, 319.
20. Pennisi, V.R. To facilitate the suitable location of the nipple in breast reduction and reconstruction. *Plast. Reconstr. Surg.* **1987**, *80*, 474. [CrossRef]
21. Pennisi, V.R.; Klabunde, E.H.; Pletsch, M.E. The location of the nipple in breast reconstruction. *Plast. Reconstr. Surg.* **1969**, *43*, 612–617. [CrossRef]
22. Laschuk, M.J.; Head, L.K.; Roumeliotis, G.A.; Xuan, L.; Silverman, H.J. The rule of thirds: Determining the ideal areolar proportions. *JPRAS Open* **2019**, *23*, 55–59. [CrossRef] [PubMed]

23. I Berson, M. Construction of pseudoareola. *Surgery* **1946**, *20*, 808. [PubMed]
24. Kristoffersen, C.M.; Seland, H.; Hansson, E. A systematic review of risks and benefits with nipple-areola-reconstruction. *J. Plast. Surg. Hand Surg.* **2016**, *51*, 1–9. [CrossRef] [PubMed]
25. Guerra, A.B.; Khoobehi, K.; Metzinger, S.E.; Allen, R.J. New Technique for Nipple Areola Reconstruction: Arrow Flap and Rib Cartilage Graft for Long-Lasting Nipple Projection. *Ann. Plast. Surg.* **2003**, *50*, 31–37. [CrossRef] [PubMed]
26. Rubino, C.; Dessy, L.A.; Posadinu, A. A modified technique for nipple reconstruction: The 'arrow flap'. *Br. J. Plast. Surg.* **2003**, *56*, 247–251. [CrossRef]
27. Jones, G.; Bostwick, J., 3rd. Nipple-Areolar Complex Reconstruction. *Nipple-Areolar Complex Reconstr.* **2018**, *1*, 35–38. [CrossRef]
28. Lewis, J.R., Jr. Reconstruction of the nipple. *Aesthetic Plast Surg.* **1980**, *4*, 311–323. [CrossRef]
29. Krogsgaard, S.H.; Carstensen, L.F.; Thomsen, J.B.; Rose, M. Nipple Reconstruction. *Plast. Reconstr. Surg. Glob. Open* **2019**, *7*, e2262. [CrossRef]
30. Vozza, A.; LaRocca, F.; Ferraro, G.; Nicoletti, F.; D'Andrea, F. The oval technique for nipple-areolar complex reconstruction. *Arch. Plast. Surg.* **2019**, *46*, 129–134. [CrossRef]
31. Few, J.W.; Marcus, J.R.; A Casas, L.; E Aitken, M.; Redding, J. Long-term predictable nipple projection following reconstruction. *Plast. Reconstr. Surg.* **1999**, *104*, 1321–1324. [CrossRef]
32. Kaplan, J.; Reece, E.; Belfort, B.; Winocour, S.J. Repeated C-V Flap for Loss of Projection in Nipple Reconstruction. *Plast. Reconstr. Surg.* **2020**, *145*, 884e–885e. [CrossRef] [PubMed]
33. Bernard, R.W.; Beran, S.J. Autologous Fat Graft in Nipple Reconstruction. *Plast. Reconstr. Surg.* **2003**, *112*, 964–968. [CrossRef] [PubMed]
34. Guerid, S.; Boucher, F.; Mojallal, A. Nipple reconstruction using rib cartilage strut in microsurgical reconstructed breast. *Annales de Chirurgie Plastique Esthétique* **2017**, *62*, 332–335. [CrossRef] [PubMed]
35. Cheng, M.-H.; Rodriguez, E.D.; Smartt, J.M.; Cardenas-Mejia, A. Nipple Reconstruction Using the Modified Top Hat Flap With Banked Costal Cartilage Graft. *Ann. Plast. Surg.* **2007**, *59*, 621–628. [CrossRef] [PubMed]
36. Cheng, M.-H.; Ho-Asjoe, M.; Wei, F.-C.; Chuang, D.C.C. Nipple reconstruction in Asian females using banked cartilage graft and modified top hat flap. *Br. J. Plast. Surg.* **2003**, *56*, 692–694. [CrossRef]
37. Heitland, A.S.; Markowicz, M.; Koellensperger, E.; Allen, R.; Pallua, N. Long-term nipple shrinkage following augmentation by an autologous rib cartilage transplant in free DIEP-flaps. *J. Plast. Reconstr. Aesthetic Surg.* **2006**, *59*, 1063–1067. [CrossRef]
38. Jones, A.P.; Erdmann, M. Projection and patient satisfaction using the "Hamburger" nipple reconstruction technique. *J. Plast. Reconstr. Aesthetic Surg.* **2012**, *65*, 207–212. [CrossRef]
39. Kurlander, D.E.; Collis, G.; Bernard, S. Autologous dermal fat graft modification for skate flap nipple reconstruction. *J. Plast. Reconstr. Aesthetic Surg.* **2016**, *69*, e44–e45. [CrossRef] [PubMed]
40. Garramone, C.E.; Lam, B. Use of AlloDerm in Primary Nipple Reconstruction to Improve Long-Term Nipple Projection. *Plast. Reconstr. Surg.* **2007**, *119*, 1663–1668. [CrossRef]
41. Colwell, A.S.; Breuing, K.H. Primary Nipple Reconstruction with AlloDerm: Is a Dermal Flap Always Necessary? *Plast. Reconstr. Surg.* **2009**, *124*, 260e–262e. [CrossRef]
42. Kim, E.K.; Lee, T.J. Use of Lyophilized Allogeneic Costal Cartilage: Is it effective to maintain the projection of the reconstructed nipple? *Ann. Plast. Surg.* **2011**, *66*, 128–130. [CrossRef] [PubMed]
43. Panettiere, P.; Marchetti, L.; Accorsi, D. Filler Injection Enhances the Projection of the Reconstructed Nipple: An Original Easy Technique. *Aesthetic Plast. Surg.* **2005**, *29*, 287–294. [CrossRef] [PubMed]
44. Evans, K.K.; Rasko, Y.; Lenert, J.; Olding, M. The use of calcium hydroxylapatite for nipple projection after failed nipple-areolar reconstruction: Early results. *Ann. Plast. Surg.* **2005**, *55*, 25–29. [CrossRef] [PubMed]
45. Sue, G.R.; Seither, J.G.; Nguyen, D. Use of hyaluronic acid filler for enhancement of nipple projection following breast reconstruction: An easy and effective technique. *JPRAS Open* **2019**, *23*, 19–25. [CrossRef] [PubMed]
46. Oliver, J.D.; Beal, C.; Hu, M.S.; Sinno, S.; Hammoudeh, Z.S. Allogeneic and Alloplastic Augmentation Grafts in Nipple–Areola Complex Reconstruction: A Systematic Review and Pooled Outcomes Analysis of Complications and Aesthetic Outcomes. *Aesthetic Plast. Surg.* **2019**, *44*, 308–314. [CrossRef] [PubMed]
47. Serre, A.; Guillier, D.; Moris, V.; Rem, K.; Revol, M.; François, C.; Cristofari, S. Nipple projection augmentation in breast reconstruction by artificial derm injection. *Annales de Chirurgie Plastique et Esthetique* **2017**, *62*, 625–629. [CrossRef]

48. Jankau, J.; Jaskiewicz, J.; Ankiewicz, A. A new method for using a silicone rod for permanent nipple projection after breast reconstruction procedures. *Breast* **2011**, *20*, 124–128. [CrossRef]
49. Tierney, B.P.; Hodde, J.P.; Changkuon, D.I. Biologic Collagen Cylinder with Skate Flap Technique for Nipple Reconstruction. *Plast. Surg. Int.* **2014**, *2014*, 194087. [CrossRef]
50. Collins, B.; Williams, J.Z.; Karu, H.; Hodde, J.P.; Martin, V.A.; Gurtner, G.C. Nipple Reconstruction with the Biodesign Nipple Reconstruction Cylinder: A Prospective Clinical Study. *Plast. Reconstr. Surg. Glob. Open* **2016**, *4*, e832. [CrossRef]
51. Chia, H.-L.; Wong, M.; Tan, B.-K. Nipple Reconstruction with Rolled Dermal Graft Support. *Arch. Plast. Surg.* **2014**, *41*, 158–162. [CrossRef]
52. Heo, J.-W.; Park, S.O.; Jin, U.S. A Nipple–Areolar Complex Reconstruction in Implant-Based Breast Reconstruction Using a Local Flap and Full-Thickness Skin Graft. *Aesthetic Plast. Surg.* **2018**, *42*, 1478–1484. [CrossRef]
53. Adams, W.M. Labial transplant for correction of loss of the nipple. *Plast. Reconstr. Surg.* **1949**, *4*, 295–298. [CrossRef] [PubMed]
54. Zenn, M.R.; Garofalo, J.A. Unilateral Nipple Reconstruction with Nipple Sharing: Time for a Second Look. *Plast. Reconstr. Surg.* **2009**, *123*, 1648–1653. [CrossRef] [PubMed]
55. Sakai, S.; Taneda, H. New Nipple-Sharing Technique That Preserves the Anatomic Structure of the Donor Nipple for Breastfeeding. *Aesthetic Plast. Surg.* **2011**, *36*, 308–312. [CrossRef] [PubMed]
56. Haslik, W.; Nedomansky, J.; Hacker, S.; Nickl, S.; Schroegendorfer, K. Objective and subjective evaluation of donor-site morbidity after nipple sharing for nipple areola reconstruction. *J. Plast. Reconstr. Aesthetic Surg.* **2015**, *68*, 168–174. [CrossRef] [PubMed]
57. Liliav, B.; Loeb, J.; Hassid, V.J.; Antony, A.K. Single-Stage Nipple-Areolar Complex Reconstruction Technique, Outcomes, and Patient Satisfaction. *Ann. Plast. Surg.* **2014**, *73*, 492–497. [CrossRef] [PubMed]
58. Spear, S.L.; Arias, J. Long-Term Experience with Nipple-Areola Tattooing. *Ann. Plast. Surg.* **1995**, *35*, 232–236. [CrossRef]
59. Uhlmann, N.R.; Martins, M.M.; Piato, S. 3D areola dermopigmentation (nipple-areola complex). *Breast J.* **2019**, *25*, 1214–1221. [CrossRef]
60. Cha, H.G.; Kwon, J.G.; Kim, E.K. Simultaneous Nipple–Areola Complex Reconstruction Technique: Combination Nipple Sharing and Tattooing. *Aesthetic Plast. Surg.* **2018**, *43*, 76–82. [CrossRef]
61. Lee, H.C.; Eom, J.S.; Kim, E.K.; Lee, T.J. Does the Sequence of Tattooing and Nipple Reconstruction Affect Nipple Projection? *Ann. Plast. Surg.* **2017**, *79*, 430–432. [CrossRef]
62. Sasaki, Y.; Matsumine, H. Modified Medical Tattooing Techniques in Nipple-areola Complex Reconstruction. *Plast. Reconstr. Surg. Glob. Open* **2018**, *6*, e1926. [CrossRef] [PubMed]
63. Cha, H.G.; Kwon, J.G.; Kim, E.K.; Lee, H.J. Tattoo-only nipple-areola complex reconstruction: Another option for plastic surgeons. *J. Plast. Reconstr. Aesthetic Surg.* **2020**, *73*, 696–702. [CrossRef] [PubMed]
64. Azouz, S.; Swanson, M.; Omarkhil, M.; Rebecca, A. A Nipple-Areola Stencil for Three-Dimensional Tattooing. *Plast. Reconstr. Surg.* **2020**, *145*, 38–42. [CrossRef] [PubMed]
65. Joseph, W.J.; Roy, E.; Stofman, G.M. Delayed Hypersensitivity Reaction after Nipple Tattooing: A Novel Case Report. *Plast. Reconstr. Surg. Glob. Open* **2019**, *7*, e2394. [CrossRef]
66. Starnoni, M.; Pinelli, M.; Franceschini, G.; De Santis, G. A Rare Case of Nipple–Areolar Complex Partial Necrosis following Micropigmentation: What to Learn? *Plast. Reconstr. Surg. Glob. Open* **2019**, *7*, e2494. [CrossRef] [PubMed]
67. Obasi, J. Micropigmentation of the nipple–areola complex after breast cancer reconstruction surgery. *Oxf. Med Case Rep.* **2019**, *2019*. [CrossRef]
68. Sainsbury, R.; Walker, V.A.; Smith, P.M. An improved nipple prosthesis. *Ann. R. Coll. Surg. Engl.* **1991**, *73*, 67–69.
69. Roberts, A.C.; Coleman, D.J.; Sharpe, D.T. Custom-made nipple-areola prostheses in breast reconstruction. *Br. J. Plast. Surg.* **1988**, *41*, 586–587. [CrossRef]
70. Ward, C.M. The uses of external nipple-areola prostheses following reconstruction of a breast mound after mastectomy. *Br. J. Plast. Surg.* **1985**, *38*, 51–54. [CrossRef]
71. Clarkson, D.; Smith, P.; Thorpe, R.; Daly, J. The use of custom-made external nipple-areolar prostheses following breast cancer reconstruction. *J. Plast. Reconstr. Aesthetic Surg.* **2011**, *64*, e103–e105. [CrossRef]
72. Ullmann, Y.; Peled, I.J.; Laufer, D.; Blumenfeld, I. Nipple-Areola Reconstruction with a Custom-made Silicone Ectoprosthesis. *Ann. Plast. Surg.* **1992**, *28*, 485–487. [CrossRef] [PubMed]

73. Hallock, G.G. Polyurethane Nipple Prosthesis. *Ann. Plast. Surg.* **1990**, *24*, 80–85. [CrossRef] [PubMed]
74. Cohen, I.K. Reconstruction of the nipple-areola by dermabrasion in a black patient. *Plast Reconstr. Surg.* **1981**, *67*, 238–239. [CrossRef] [PubMed]
75. De Cholnoky, T. Breast reconstruction after radical mastectomy: Formation of missing nipple by everted navel. *Plast. Reconstr. Surg.* **1966**, *38*. [CrossRef] [PubMed]
76. Ishii, N.; Ando, J.; Harao, M.; Takemae, M.; Kishi, K. Influence of Flap Thickness on Nipple Projection after Nipple Reconstruction Using a Modified Star Flap. *Aesthetic Plast. Surg.* **2018**, *42*, 964–970. [CrossRef]
77. Satteson, E.S.; Reynolds, M.F.; Bond, A.M.; Pestana, I.A. An Analysis of Complication Risk Factors in 641 Nipple Reconstructions. *Breast J.* **2016**, *22*, 379–383. [CrossRef] [PubMed]
78. Pizzonia, G.; Sasso, A.; Rossello, C. Alternative technique for nipple-areola complex reconstruction with poor skin condition. *ANZ J. Surg.* **2015**, *87*. [CrossRef]

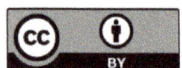

© 2020 by the author. Licensee MDPI, Basel, Switzerland. This article is an open access article distributed under the terms and conditions of the Creative Commons Attribution (CC BY) license (http://creativecommons.org/licenses/by/4.0/).

MDPI
St. Alban-Anlage 66
4052 Basel
Switzerland
Tel. +41 61 683 77 34
Fax +41 61 302 89 18
www.mdpi.com

Medicina Editorial Office
E-mail: medicina@mdpi.com
www.mdpi.com/journal/medicina

www.ingramcontent.com/pod-product-compliance
Lightning Source LLC
LaVergne TN
LVHW070542100526
838202LV00012B/350